Medication Management in Care of Older People

Medication Management in Care of Older People

Edited by
Dr Maggi Banning

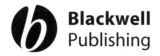
Blackwell
Publishing

Editorial offices:
Blackwell Publishing Ltd, 9600 Garsington Road, Oxford OX4 2DQ, UK
Tel: +44 (0)1865 776868
Blackwell Publishing Inc., 350 Main Street, Malden, MA 02148-5020, USA
Tel: +1 781 388 8250
Blackwell Publishing Asia Pty Ltd, 550 Swanston Street, Carlton, Victoria
3053, Australia
Tel: +61 (0)3 8359 1011

First published 2007 by Blackwell Publishing Ltd

ISBN: 978-1-4051-5174-0

Library of Congress Cataloging-in-Publication Data

Medication management in care of older people / edited by Maggi Banning.
p. ; cm.
Includes bibliographical references and index.
ISBN-13: 978-1-4051-5174-0 (pbk. : alk. paper)
ISBN-10: 1-4051-5174-9 (pbk. : alk. paper)
1. Geriatric pharmacology–Great Britain. 2. Older people–Drug use–Great
Britain. 3. Medication abuse–Great Britain–Prevention. I. Banning, Maggi.
[DNLM: 1. Aged. 2. Drug Therapy–methods. 3. Medication Errors–
prevention & control. 4. Medication Systems–organization &
administration. 5. Patient Care Planning. 6. Pharmaceutical Services. WT
166 M4886 2007]

RC953.7.M42 2007
615.5′80846–dc22
2007000572

A catalogue record for this title is available from the British Library
Set in 10/12 pt Palatino
by SNP Best-set Typesetter Ltd., Hong Kong
Printed and bound in Singapore
by COS Printers Pte Ltd

The publisher's policy is to use permanent paper from mills that operate a
sustainable forestry policy, and which has been manufactured from pulp
processed using acid-free and elementary chlorine-free practices. Furthermore, the publisher ensures that the text paper and cover board used have
met acceptable environmental accreditation standards.

For further information on Blackwell Publishing, visit our website:
www.blackwellpublishing.com

Contents

List of figures

List of tables

About the contributors

Maggi Banning, EdD, MSc, PGDE, BSc, SRN, SCM, is a Senior Lecturer at Brunel University where she is division director for Health Studies and Community Health. She teaches applied research to undergraduate and postgraduate students studying for qualifications in community health, as well as applied research, teaching and learning to undergraduate students studying for a BSc in Health Studies. She also teaches applied pharmacology to health visitors studying for a nurse prescribing qualification.

Dr Andy Evenden, PhD, BSc, is Principal Lecturer in Biomedical Sciences in the School of Biological Sciences at the University of Plymouth. Since 1997 he has taught biomedical sciences to students of the health care professions, medicine and human biosciences. Andy is a recipient of a University of Plymouth Teaching Fellowship as well as an Innovation Fellowship from the University's Centre for Excellence in Professional Placement Learning. Andy has research interests that involve teaching and learning strategies for integration of biomedicine into health care, and the educational engagement of students with 'non-biological' backgrounds.

Karen Gesty, PhD, BSc, is Principal Lecturer in Biological Aspects of Health in the School of Biological Sciences at the University of Plymouth. She has taught human biology to health professional and science students since 1995, with a particular interest in teaching the subject to non-biologists. Karen has been awarded a University of Plymouth Teaching Fellowship as well as an Innovation Fellowship from the University's Centre for Excellence in Professional Placement Learning. Her particular research interests are centred on educational e-support for health care students in the subject of biosciences, as well as public communication and engagement with science.

Cliff Roberts, PhD, MSc, BSc, SRN, is Senior Lecturer in Science at London South Bank University, Post Registration Nursing Dept. His clinical specialism lies in physiology, pathophysiology and pharmacology in Clinical Neuroscience and Psychobiology. His research interests focus on experimental studies on the effects of stress on changes in mental health, eating behaviour and body weight. Dissemination of this research is through international conference presentations and publications.

Jon Waterfield, BPharm, MSc (Pharmacology), MRPharmS, PGCE, is Senior Lecturer in Pharmacy Practice and Clinical Pharmacy at Leicester School of Pharmacy, De Montfort University. Jon registered as a pharmacist in 1984 and has worked mainly in community pharmacy, education and training. For several years he was Pharmacy Training Manager for Lloydspharmacy. As a community pharmacist he has been extensively involved in medicines management services to residential and nursing homes for older people. In his current role Jon is Pre-registration Tutor for Leicester School of Pharmacy and is mainly involved in delivering pharmacy practice teaching to undergraduates. He is currently writing a book on community pharmacy due to be published in 2008.

Tracy Wills, BSc, MSc, DE, RGN, is a Senior Lecturer at De Montfort University Leicester where she teaches on the Pre-registration Nursing course in the primary care field and is the Pathway leader for BSc (Hons) specialist community health nursing in District Nursing. She has been a practice development nurse across several community hospitals in the past, a community practice teacher and a district nurse for many years. Her interest in contributing to this book was her concern for older people in managing their medication in the community, with particular reference to the timely and accurate administration of medication and the patients' difficulties in managing multiple medications.

Preface

This book is intended for health care professionals who either have an interest in medication management and older people, or are qualified independent or supplementary prescribers. This introductory text is designed to provide an overview of the issues and knowledge and clinical relevance relevant to the medication management of older people. The book includes chapters that discuss the biology and neurobiology of ageing, pathological conditions such as Parkinson's and Alzheimer's disease, and the principles of applied pharmacology and its relationship to older people. Towards the end of the book there are profession-specific chapters relevant to nurses, community matrons and pharmacists.

The idea and motivation for the book came initially from my experience of teaching applied pharmacology to qualified nurses and professionals studying to become independent and supplementary prescribers, but also from my interest in prescribing for older people. This book is aimed at giving qualified health care professionals and students an introduction to the influential factors that have a direct impact on medicines management, with specific emphasis on older people.

The layout of this book is straightforward and each chapter can be read on its own without the need to continually refer to other chapters. Each chapter has learning outcomes and implications for practice; references to publications referred to in each chapter can be found towards the end of the book.

We hope that this book will make medication management interesting for health care practitioners and will stimulate further exploration of the subject. More importantly, our desire is to see health care practitioners comprehend the principles of applied pharmacology and medication management to enable them to use this knowledge in their daily practice.

Introduction

Maggi Banning

The focus of this book is to introduce the reader to the concept of medication management and its importance to older people. Medication management is a broad term that encompasses patient-centred medication review, the single assessment process, rational prescribing, access to medicines, improvements at the primary/secondary care interface, repeat prescribing and the identification of the adverse effects of medicines (Medicines Partnership, 2002). Medication mismanagement occurs when patients fail to administer their medicines in the manner prescribed by the physician/nurse or pharmacist prescriber. The mismanagement of medicines is a significant problem and can be a contributing factor in the development of drug-induced iatrogenic disease. In addition, older people are prone to additional health risks associated with increasing age such as physical debilitation and forgetfulness, both of which can directly predispose them to mismanage their medicines.

In 1989, the Department of Health and the Welsh Office issued guidelines for monitoring individuals over the age of 75 years, in the form of an annual health check. Older people were identified as a group of individuals who were vulnerable, and required review of medication and exploration for iatrogenic disease. The need for this procedure arose as a consequence of the increased potential for chronic disease states, iatrogenic disease, adverse effects developing from prescribed medication and medication mismanagement in elderly patients (Lindley & Tulley, 1992) and because older people are more sensitive to the actions of medicines (RCP, 1997). This recognition led to strategic initiatives that centred on the increased surveillance of older people as illustrated in the National Service Framework for Older People (DoH, 2001).

Each of the nine chapters in this book introduces concepts of medicines management that are pertinent to the management of older people and their medicines.

Since the year 2000, the British Government has been committed to modernising the National Health Service (NHS) through a series of patient-centred health policies and improved health education and training schemes. The central goal of government policy is to use the knowledge, skills and experience of health care professionals such as nurses, pharmacists and allied health care professionals to enhance the quality of patient care and the provision of services to the general public. A central feature of these policies is the provision of further education and training for health care professionals in medication management, applied pharmacology and therapeutics and physical assessment and prescribing practice. Added to this is the importance of developing initiatives to provide both health care and social services to older people. Older people are specifically targeted because of their medication management needs and the impact that this has on essential services such as GPs, hospitals and community nurses.

The aim of Chapter 1 is to explore the key influential government documents that have shaped the development and implementation of health care policy since the year 2000. This chapter also examines issues and problems related to the prescribing, dispensing and administration of medicines by professionals and patients, and introduces the community matron's role and its impact on the health and medicines management of older people with long-term conditions. It provides an overview of the medication management partnership scheme and explores medication management issues using a case study that illustrates how medicines impact on a patient's life.

Ageing is a constant process that can commence from a very early age, for example atherosclerotic changes in arteries have been found in children as young as 6 years old. The biology of ageing involves the complex interplay between physiological and biochemical changes that leads to alterations in pathophysiology which later manifest themselves in adaptations at an organ, tissue and cellular level. The aim of Chapter 2 is to describe the physiological changes that occur at all levels of biological organisation during ageing, to consider clinically relevant changes that occur during ageing and to evaluate the impact of key effects of ageing on physiological systems such as the cardiovascular and hepatic systems and changes to hepatic blood, the renal system and the effect on fluid and electrolytes and the immune system and pro-inflammatory responses.

Pharmacology is the study of drugs and their use in the treatment of pathological conditions. To understand the principles of pharmacology, it is essential that the individual understands the basic principles of applied physiology and pathophysiology at all levels of biological organisation. Knowledge in these scientific subjects forms the basis of comprehending how drugs work and how the body responds to them. Both elements are essential to prescribing medicines and developing expertise in medication management. In Chapter 3, the reader is introduced to the basic principles of pharmacology: pharmacokinetics and pharmacodynamics. The chapter commences with an overview of pharmacokinetic principles and discusses the impact of ageing on drug absorption, drug distribution, drug metabolism and drug excretion. This is followed by an introduction to the modes of action of drugs and the influence of ageing on drug sensitivity. The chapter concludes with an introduction to performance indicators and how they can be used as a measure of appropriate prescribing of medicines for older people.

According to the National Pharmaceutical Association, medication management is everyone's problem. It is a concept that infiltrates every household and every family at some point in their lives. Medication management is a multi-factorial process that is dependent on the pharmacovigilance of the prescriber. In order to tackle the problems of medication management in the older person, an educational programme was developed that centred on the single assessment process and the use of trigger questions to screen older people and their medication and social care needs. Pharmacists and nurses underwent additional education and training in order to become single assessment process assessors. A series of four trigger questions was developed to assess the extent to which older people are concordant with their medication. The single assessment process is a tiered process which can involve other members of the health care team dependent on the health and social care that the older person requires. Chapter 4 provides an introduction to the concept of medication management with particular attention paid to the needs of older people. This is followed by discussion on the need for patient-centred medication review and the importance of the single assessment process and associated trigger questions. The principles of prescribing will be introduced in addition to the concept of rational prescribing and prescribing support in relation to older people. These topics are extremely relevant to both the prescriber and the community matron who care for older people and manage their medicines.

Medication errors are a global concern that can be costly in terms of the financial costs, but also because of the potential detrimental influences on the physical health of older people. Older people are prone to the adverse consequences of drugs due to their increased sensitivity to the actions of medicine. This sensitivity is increased when errors occur involving the prescription, dispensing or supply and administration of drugs. Chapter 5 will examine the concept of medication errors and their impact on older people. The chapter commences with an overview of the global prevalence of medication errors, an introduction to the system that is used to classify medication errors, and an exploration of the aetiology and underpinning causes of medication errors. This is followed by an examination of the factors associated with medication errors that arise owing to the administration and supply of medicines. The final section of this chapter includes an introduction to preventative measures that can be taken to reduce the development of medication errors that arise due to the supply and administration of medicines or associated with nurse prescribing.

As people get older their physiological systems begin to malfunction and as a consequence of this malfunctioning, pathophysiological conditions develop. In many cases, several pathophysiological conditions may develop concurrently, each requiring pharmacological management. This factor augments the risk of polypharmacy which may account for the growing costs of medical care in the UK. It is estimated that up to 45% of the medicines prescribed in the UK are prescribed for older people. This figure is set to increase with the quantitative rise in number of people over the age of 65 years in the UK. In 2002, the Office for National Statistics reported that 18.6% of the population is over the age of 65 years; this is thought to rise to more than 20% by the year 2010. As people get older they can become socially and physically vulnerable, which is augmented by memory loss, incipient dementia and physical weakness. These factors can lead to problems associated with concordance with medication. Chapter 6 explores the concept of concordance, underpinning features of concordance, and factors and relevant research pertinent to medication-taking behaviour. This chapter also explores the role of the nurse in the prevention of non-concordant behaviour, with an examination of measures that can be used to promote patient education in an attempt to improve concordance with medication.

As part of the ageing process, a considerable number of older people will develop neurophysiological problems such as Alzheimer's disease, senile dementia and depression. These conditions are often associated with impaired cerebral functions such as loss of long-term and short-term memory, sleep disorders and mood and behavioural changes. The aim of Chapter 7 is to provide an overview of neurophysiology, a short history of drug development in relation to the treatment of neurophysiological conditions and an exploration of common neurophysiological problems that affect older people, with an overview of the possible treatment options available.

As the number of older people with pre-existing long-term conditions rises, there is an associated increase in the demand for improved health care and social services. With an increasingly older population, the risk of medication mismanagement and iatrogenic disease due to polypharmacy augments the quantity of unplanned admission to hospital. The current government is committed to reducing the quantity of unplanned admissions to hospital for people with long-term conditions through the development and implementation of the community matron's role. Throughout England, an education and training programme was implemented to educate and train senior nurses to take on advanced practice roles in case management and to provide quality health and social care for patients with long-term conditions. This education and training programme is commensurate with the Government's Knowledge and Skills Framework and the principles of advanced practice as outlined by the Nursing and Midwifery Council (NMC).

The aim of Chapter 8 is to explore the government's policy for England with respect to the management of patients with long-term conditions, in particular older people. The chapter explores current developments with respect to National Service Framework (NSF) for Older People, the NHS Improvement Plan, the education and training of the community matron, the role of lay carer in the management of older people and their medicines, and future developments with respect to the education and training of community matrons and nurse prescribers.

Since 2000, the role of the community pharmacist in the medication management of older people has evolved. Currently, many community pharmacists work collaboratively with community matrons and GPs to monitor the management of older people and their medicines, and also undertake prescribing and medication assessment roles. The aim of Chapter 9 is to provide an overview of the role of the community pharmacist in the management of older people and their medicines. The chapter will commence with an introduction to the education and training of pharmacists, followed by an assessment of the community pharmacist contractual framework, exploration of initiatives such as repeat prescribing, medicines-use reviews with illustrations of specific drugs and common problems regarding their use. The chapter will also explore pharmacy-driven services such as medication review, domiciliary visiting and residential homes schemes, and prescribing support for older people who may suffer from falls, stroke or mental health problems. The latter part of the chapter examines issues such as how to manage patients with swallowing difficulties, provision of compliance aids, and the need for multi-disciplinary working and pharmacy services.

Overall, this book aims to introduce the reader to the concept of medication management specific to older people. For many nurses medication management may be a term that they relate to nurse prescribing. However, it could be argued that it is a process that is pertinent to the holistic management of patients and their conditions and should be an essential component of nurse education as it crosses the boundaries of primary and secondary care. For effective medicines management, all health care professionals involved in the management of older people and their medicines need to possess a comprehensive knowledge of applied pharmacology and therapeutics, and issues related to the concordance of medication.

Older people and their medicines: health objectives and health initiatives

Tracy Wills

Learning objectives

The aim of this chapter is to explore current government objectives and initiatives that have influenced the management of medicines in older people. This will centre on the following:

- an overview of the key influential government documents
- consideration of errors in prescribing, dispensing and administration of medicines
- examples of good practice influenced by government initiatives that improve medicines management of older people
- the community matron's role and its impact on the health and medicines management of older people with long term conditions
- a case study demonstrating how medicines impact on a patient's life, indicating areas that require improvement as indicated by the government initiatives.

Introduction

The main service users of health and social provision are older people. In 1998–1999 40% of the National Health Service (NHS) budget was spent on people aged over 65 years in England (DoH, 2001). Between the years 2000 and 2004 there was a 16% rise in the number of hours of home care provided, with a 27% rise in intensive home care hours

(DoH, 2000a, 2004c). It is recognised in today's society that older people are a valuable resource rather than a burden; therefore we should ensure optimum health in this client group. Long-term conditions affect predominantly older people, particularly those in lower socio-economic groups, therefore good quality personal support services are needed to enable this group to manage their own treatment effectively and slow disease progression, thus avoiding emergency admissions to hospital (DoH, 2004c).

In a press release in January 2005, the then Health Secretary, John Reid, announced a major overhaul in the way health and social care services deliver care to the millions of people in England with long-term conditions. Long-term conditions are those conditions that cannot be cured, but can be controlled by medication and other therapies (Beasley, 2005).

Development of the National Service Framework (NSF) for Older People

The Department of Health (DoH) states that 'people expect the NHS to treat them when they are ill and view health as the responsibility of the doctor' (DoH, 2004c, p. 48). Generally older people tend to expect less service provision than younger age groups. Consequently older people have not always been high on the list of priorities in terms of service provision tailored to meet their specific needs. However, the inception of the NSF for Older People (DoH, 2001) attempts to address this with a 10-year plan for improving the quality of health and social care for the older person; indeed standard 1 is rooting out age discrimination.

The DoH recognises that organisational structures can be a barrier to the assessment of need and access to care, and proposes better integration of health and social care services through the use of the single assessment process (Milburn, 2001). The single assessment process results in improvement in the sharing of information and resources and in medication use, more specifically to question (DoH, 2001c, 2004a):

- How do patients obtain their medication?
- Can the patient read the label, open containers and swallow tablets with ease?
- Do they think the medication could work better?
- Do patients take their medication as prescribed?

It is estimated that around 50% of patients on long-term medication do not take it as prescribed (DoH 2001c, 2005b).

There are several standards mentioned in the NSF that are worth discussing. Standard 2 relates to informed choices that older people should be offered, e.g. benefit versus side effects with their medication.

The patient should be allowed to determine their own level of acceptable risk. In order to achieve this, patients and their carers need to understand the level of care that needs to be provided and know who to contact if a problem arises (DoH, 2001). Standard 4 relates to the need for older people managed in hospital to receive good medicines management and pain control that is underpinned by an assessment of functional capability. Standard 5 relates to the identification of high-risk groups and application of medical interventions with the aim of preventing strokes. Stroke patients usually administer a combination of preventative medicines, such as aspirin, warfarin and antihypertensive medications, which require regular medication reviews to facilitate concordance and avoid the complications of polypharmacy.

NSF Standard 6 is important as it relates to the identification of intrinsic risk factors pertinent to the development of falls; these include polypharmacy (administering four or more drugs concurrently), particularly sedating and antihypertensive therapies, and the quantity of falls. A person who has these characteristics will be referred to a dedicated falls service. An individual from the team will then review the suitability of the patient's medication, discontinue or change medications to more suitable options and also consider the addition of vitamin D and calcium supplements to high-risk patients (DoH, 2001a).

Management of medicines

In 2004, the DoH published a white paper as a resource to support the implementation of the wider aspects of medicines management for the NSFs for Diabetes, Renal Services and Long-term Conditions (DoH, 2004a), as previously recommended in 'Medicines and Older People' (DoH, 2001c). Although the number of dedicated NSFs is limited, the NSF for Long-term Conditions can be widely applied to older people with long-term illness.

The DoH defines medicines management as 'the clinical, cost effective and safe use of medicines to ensure that patients get the maximum benefit from the medicines they need, while at the same time minimising potential harm' (DoH, 2004a, p. 1). The underpinning values inherent in the medicines management resource document (DoH, 2004a) are that the patient is a partner and has choices in any decision making about their medicines, and that all patients and their carers have equal and improved access to medicines and related information. With training, the patient is the best person to manage their own condition. This concept is underpinned by the expert patient programmes recommended by the DoH in 2002. The resource document also encourages professionals to expand the role boundaries and work collaboratively to support the patient in holistic management of their own condition (DoH, 2004a).

Professionals have access to current evidence through the National Institute for Health and Clinical Excellence (NICE, 2002) but since 2005 there was little NHS provision to prepare patients to access the relevant information independently in order to achieve effective self management; for example, the NHS Direct Online, the electronic Medicines Compendium or PRODIGY patient information leaflets.

The NHS Improvement Plan

Improving health services patient safety is paramount, and risk reduction is a key issue on the government agenda. To achieve this, the DoH (2004c) aims to extend the expert patients programmes by 2008. The aim of this programme is to educate patients in the management of their own condition and to raise awareness of possible problems in purchasing over the counter and complementary therapy medicines. In practice, many patients do not discuss medicines that have been purchased from complementary therapists or over the counter in supermarkets or health food shops. These medicines will not appear on their medication record. Contra-indications may go undetected; for example, St John's wort, widely available to purchase and taken for depression, limits the effectiveness of warfarin and indinavir used in HIV therapies and cyclosporine (National Centre for Complementary and Alternative Medicine, 2004). To address this problem, the NHS Improvement Plan (DoH, 2004c) supports the Health Protection Agency in proposals to regulate complementary therapists.

The DoH recognises that a person's medicine should be only a small part of their life in terms of physical, social and psychological well-being, but it has the potential to take over as the main life focus in these areas if not effectively managed (DoH, 2004c). As a result of this, a key role of the NHS Improvement Plan (DoH, 2004c) is to integrate the provision of health and social care for patients that require these services through social care commissioning. This will improve the management of resources, e.g. a patient that needs help, such as prompting, with medicines. In the past this has been a grey area between health and social care, which has now been addressed by government initiatives.

Building a Safer NHS for Patients; the role of medication safety

The aim of the report Building a Safer NHS for Patients, by the chief pharmaceutical officer at the DoH, is to 'embed a culture of safety in all NHS treatment . . . ensuring that drug treatment is safe' (DoH, 2004b). A 40% reduction in serious errors relating to prescribed drugs is anticipated.

Learning from mistakes and altering practice and procedures in the light of that learning (An Organisation with a Memory – DOH, 2000b) is the underpinning ideology of the National Patient Safety Agency (NPSA) established by government. To keep the level of drug errors in perspective, the DoH (2004) reports that of 660 million prescriptions written by GPs annually, less than 1% had claims against them for prescribing errors or for pharmacists' dispensing errors. This does not account for errors made in administration of medicines by professionals or patients themselves, nor does it account for errors where no claim was made. No one involved in prescribing, dispensing or administration of medicines can afford to be complacent.

The following section considers where mistakes in prescribing, dispensing and administration of medicines by professionals to patients are commonly made.

Prescribing drugs

The process of drug prescribing may be adversely affected by the following:

* inadequate knowledge of drug or patient's clinical condition
* calculation mistakes
* confusion of drug names.

Repeat prescribing, although often convenient for the patient, is not without its problems. Tulip and Campbell (2001) found that for each patient reviewed, at least one drug was inappropriate. In one GP practice, 66% of patients were given repeat prescriptions that were unauthorised by a doctor and 72% of patients had not had a medication review in 15 months (Zermansky, 1996). This practice is not uncommon; requests for repeat prescriptions are often managed by GP receptionists who should have robust procedures in place and receive training (DoH, 2001c, 2004).

The computerised repeat prescribing support system has supported the improvement of repeat prescribing systems by linking repeat prescribing with regular review alerts. The DoH (2001c) sets out guidance as to what this review should contain.

The introduction of the National Programme for Information Technology (NPfIT) in the NHS will utilise the NHS national electronic care record envisaged in the document Delivering the NHS Plan (DoH, 2002) and will enable health care professionals to access patients' clinical and medication details from any site. Patients will have their own 'health space' to record pertinent issues. However, information technology is only as good as the people that use it. The information must be kept up to date with back-up support systems available. In addition, there is a risk that drugs with similar names (which may or may not have a similar purpose) will appear next to each other in electronic prescribing formats; a mistake is only one click away! No amount of computer technology can replace clinical judgement or skills.

The NPfIT will be particularly pertinent in primary care when patients are admitted to care homes; in cases where the patient is either discharged from hospital to a care home or changes GP, care home staff may request prescriptions before the medical notes have transferred to the new GP, which increases the potential for prescription errors.

In 2005 e-prescribing was slowly phased in, in England, enabling easier and up-to-date repeat prescription requests. Prescriptions can be transmitted from GP direct to the community pharmacist, thus hopefully reducing prescribing errors and enabling a record of the prescription to automatically become part of the health record (DoH, 2004c, 2006). It is anticipated that this facility will be available to all GP surgery prescribers and community pharmacists by 2007, and then extended to include walk-in centres, dentists and hospitals. The Electronic Prescription Service (EPS) will form part of the new contractual framework for community pharmacists agreed between the DoH, the Pharmaceutical Services Negotiating Committee (PSNC) and the NHS Confederation (DoH, 2006).

The DoH (2004c) identifies that for patients to be empowered, they need to have the necessary skills to access, understand and use information. Access to electronic health records by patients and health professionals may not be possible in the patients' own homes unless Internet access is available. Many older people do not have or want Internet access, sometimes because they cannot afford it or understand it. There are training courses available for older people in computer skills, but again this group of people often has limitations imposed by illness and possibly finance.

Dispensing medicines

The process of dispensing may be affected by the following:

- inability to read the prescription
- confusion over the drug name
- similar packaging for different drugs
- lack of checking by a second person.

There are many occasions when a repeat prescription is requested but only one or two items on the prescription are actually required by the patient, resulting in stockpiling and wastage. The DoH (2004a) proposes that pharmacists who offer a repeat dispensing service will collect the prescription from the surgery and contact the patient to check that all items are required. For example:

- Medication such as analgesics may be prescribed 6 hourly but the patient takes them 'as required'.
- The patient has decided not to take a drug on the repeat prescription due to lifestyle/side effects or beliefs and attitudes.

Pharmacist contact with the patient prior to dispensing is also an opportunity for the pharmacist to check that there are no current problems with medication before ordering the medicines and subsequently dispensing them. These actions both save time for the patient and maintain contact with the community pharmacist, thus avoiding the dispensing of medicines that are not required. In many cases, as more pharmacists become extended prescribers and receive specific disease management training, they will be well placed to manage holistically patients' medicines, including regular reviews.

It is worth considering the difficulties that patients may have reading and understanding the label on medicines, and also whether they can open the bottle (DoH, 2004a). Several initiatives are proposed; for example, describing the condition the medicine is for on the medication label and tailoring print size to patient needs. In addition, it is noteworthy that pharmacists are obliged to provide any loose tablets in childproof containers unless otherwise requested by the patient; health professionals should ensure patients are aware of this.

The Royal Pharmaceutical Society of Great Britain suggests mnemonic 'Help' to help avoid dispensing errors (DoH, 2004). Table 1.1 shows how this translates for the pharmacy, and how it can be adapted for patients.

The author suggests the use of the mnemonic 'eeyores' as a simplified checklist, relating to the table, for patients on receipt of their medicines. This translates to Enough? Expiry date? Yours? Over-the-counter medicines? Read leaflet? Eating and drinking warnings? Side effects?

Access to medicines out of hours

Access to medicines out of hours can be a problem for older patients and has been alluded to in 'Raising standards for patients: new partnerships in out of hours care' (DoH, 2000a). The key suggestion is that prescription medicines should be available at the same time and location as the out-of-hour medical services. This is particularly difficult for older people living alone who require home visits out of hours from GPs.

The administration of drugs

Factors that influence the administration of medicines include:

- forgetfulness
- inattention

- lack of motivation
- distraction
- fatigue
- stress
- lifestyle – changing times that medicines are administered to accommodate outdoor activities.

If trained professionals can make mistakes due to the reasons cited here, so can patients or carers as they are not trained in pharmacology or medicine administration and do not always have anyone to check the medicines; but more importantly the older person on medication often suffers from ill health, fatigue and diminishing eyesight and has difficulties differentiating the similarities of packaging. The older person may not realise that they have received the wrong medicines at the prescribing or dispensing stage (DoH, 2004).

Around 80% of medications are issued in the community setting and taken by patients in their own homes or in care homes. The patient who lives in a care home often has their medication administered by untrained personnel and the medication is often stored incorrectly. The DoH (2004) cites that medicines are often kept in cluttered, untidy and

Table 1.1 Avoiding dispensing errors.

Pharmacy	Adapted for patients
How much has been dispensed	Do you have enough for the month? Did you get the full amount prescribed or does the pharmacist 'owe' you any?
Expiry date check	How long is it since you collected it? Do you know where to find the expiry date on the package? Highlight the expiry date on the package.
Label checks for correct patient name, drug name, dose and warnings	Can you see your name on the label? Does the drug name look familiar to you? If you're not sure, ring your pharmacist (some drugs have similar names but are not the same drug). Do you know what to look out for? Did you tell the prescriber or pharmacist of any medicines you take that you bought over the counter? *Read* the leaflet that came with the drugs and highlight any points that affect you. Discuss them with whoever prescribed the drugs. Is there anything you should not eat or drink with these drugs? For example, alcohol. Some side effects are merely a nuisance, others can be serious.
Product check – correct drug/dose/strength	Is the dose the same as before?

crowded storage facilities, which can be a contributory factor in administration errors; this is often the case in small residential homes or indeed the patient's bedside drawer!

The DoH (2003), in accordance with section 23 of the Care Standards Act 2000, set requirements for anyone administering medication in a care setting to have policies and procedures in place and training in safe handling and administration of medicines, including record keeping. Training must be accredited and include basic knowledge in medicine use and recognising problems and how to deal with them. Only properly labelled medicines may be given, and checking by a second person is performed (this may be the patient or carer).

Helping patients and carers to safely self-administer medicines at home or in care homes

There are several good examples of innovative practice specific to drug administration, including the following:

1. *Avoidance of administration errors using monitored dosage systems.*
Assuming that prescribing and dispensing issues are addressed, the administration of medicines by the patient or carer at home or in residential care remains a procedure that poses both difficulties and risks. Monitored dosage systems (MDS) are becoming more prominent in care homes where community pharmacists dispense all of the patient's medication into blister packs divided into day of week and time of day. There is a printed label on the back detailing drug, dose, frequency, route and expiry date, and this can be used in care homes with a printed medication administration record. These charts are not normally preprinted with patient, drug, time, dose or route and are reliant on staff accurately transposing this information. However, it can be difficult to determine which drug is which in the MDS when a patient declines some of the medication or drops it. Clearly this system is only suitable for tablets; some older people prefer dispersible or liquid forms. The MDS is useful for community nurses who may be monitoring a patient's compliance with a particular drug regime, but again it can be difficult to determine with certainty which drug is omitted.

Less formal dosage systems can be bought from chemists and supermarkets but the onus is on the patient, carers and health care staff to dispense accurately from original containers into the system. There are no information labels on these systems other than day and time.

2. *Improving knowledge and support for patients in medication management.*
There are areas of good practice in medicine management across the country; for example, in East Kent & Coastal Primary Care Trust (PCT)

there is a dedicated prescribing team to whom any member of the multi-disciplinary team may refer. They aim to assess and evaluate patient's medicines management difficulties and offer solutions, thus reducing hospital admission and care home admissions. The DoH (2004a) management of medicines resource pack offers examples of innovative practice that could be replicated and a variety of tools to assess both locality effectiveness and individual patients' efficacy in management of their own medicines.

Safwat and Goodyer (2005) studied 122 elderly patients being discharged from hospital following an intervention involving a hospital liaison pharmacist. The intervention involved counselling patients on their medication prior to discharge and then reviewing them at home up to six weeks later. During the study, liaison between the research team, the patients, the GP and the community pharmacist was maintained. Common problems identified at the six-week review were: adverse drug reactions, interactions, regimen issues, interface problems and medication storage. Further counselling was given and all details of discharge regime were communicated to the GP and community pharmacist. Although compliance and medication knowledge were found to be higher in the group receiving this intervention, there were no significant changes in the rate of hospital readmission. Although this study was hospital pharmacy based, it does support the notion that a well-informed patient is more likely to be compliant and concordant in medicine management.

3.   Improving knowledge and support for patients in medication management through regular reviews.
The Medicines Management Collaborative managed by the National Prescribing Centre has piloted initiatives to improve advice and support to patients regarding medicines management. The Task Force on Medicines Partnership was a two-year pilot project that commenced in 2003 and was supported by the DoH and the Royal Pharmaceutical Society of Great Britain. It involved a multi-professional taskforce. The focus was on putting the principles of concordance into action and integrating this approach throughout health care. The expectations were that prescribing decisions were made in agreement with patients who have come to expect this level of involvement. Resources were made available to enable the patient to do so, particularly through education. Regular medication review was cited as a fundamental requirement, as was communication between professionals and patients to achieve concordance (DoH, 2001c). In practice, GPs and pharmacists work collaboratively to regularly review patient's medication in individual reviews (DoH, 2005b). In this respect community pharmacists undertake diagnostic tests, patient education and medication review (DoH, 2005b).

The Medicines Partnership continues with alternative funding and has five key themes: professional development, good practice, health policy, research and development and communication. The partnership supports innovations that facilitate improvement in patient's medicine management, including training, shared learning and ways to get information that augments patient concordance with medication.

4.   *Prompting older people to administer their medicines.*
A project in the north-west of England targets older people and prompts them to take their medicines. This is a common problem encountered by many nurses and social carers involved in the medication management of older people. Administration of medication is a nurse's role, while prompting can be performed by a carer, but neither group have the resources to visit four to five times a day. Such a problem can be tackled using assistive technology. This process has been successfully used in America and it enables patients to remain independent in their homes (Kelham, 2005). Once a patient risk or problem is identified, the patient will have an assessment of medicines management needs by a community pharmacist who will discuss ways of managing the patient's medicines. If solutions of the traditional kind, e.g. medication management devices like the MDS, are not appropriate, an assisted technology system such as the Medicine Reminder Initiative can be ordered. This is an electronic prompting device that is connected to an existing call centre run by the patient's housing provider. The patient receives an audio and visual prompt at the time the medicine is due and the patient acknowledges the call. If no response is received the call centre mobilises services to determine if the patient is having difficulty. All disciplines involved, including call centre staff, will have received education on medicines management. The project is closely linked to social services and the anticipated outcomes are improved patient empowerment, patients have their concerns listened to and to some extent carers are relieved, and most importantly patients stay in their own home. Less time will be spent by health and social care prompting medication, and medicine-related emergencies can be averted (Kelham, 2005).
The work of the Medicines Partnership continues in collaboration with the National Prescribing Centre through external income generation. The operational plan and other initiatives can be viewed on the website http://www.medicines-partnership.org.

5.   *Implementation of health care initiatives; empowering and supporting patients in self-management of medicines.*
The American EverCare model of case management has been implemented in the UK at nine PCT pilot sites. This model includes medical and nursing assessment, including medicines management. The EverCare model focuses on proactivity and prevention to improve

quality of life and maximum independence for patients. Patients and their families are participants in care decisions, not recipients of care. The relationship between a patient and their community matron is lifelong and continuous, with varying levels of contact dependent on the stability of the patient's condition; these practitioners straddle primary, secondary and tertiary care to provide a seamless, integrated service (Redfearn & Ross, 2006).

Community matrons and the management of medicines

The concept of community matrons (CMs) evolved from the NHS Improvement Plan (DoH, 2004c) and is detailed in Supporting People with Long Term Conditions; Liberating the Talents of Nurses Who Care for People with Long Term Conditions (DoH, 2005a,b). The aim of the role is to provide a personalised service that meets the needs of patients and their carers. The CM will be responsible for and manage a case load of patients who have three or more long-term health conditions, or complex health needs, and will co-ordinate input from all of the appropriate agencies in order to manage existing problems and prevent additional problems from occurring (DoH, 2005a,b). In addition, the CM will select and refer patients to the most appropriate agency as a provider and procurer of care for those patients who require help, particularly with medicines. A key motive behind the role of the CM is to reduce the quantity of unplanned hospital admissions in patients who suffer from long-term conditions (DoH, 2005a).

The DoH (2004c) anticipates that by 2008 there will be 3000 CMs case managing 250,000 complex needs patients. Case management will include medication review and prescribing via the independent prescribing route or supplementary prescribing against an agreed management plan with the GP. Provision of education and pertinent information on aspects of the patient's medicines aims to enhance concordance.

The DoH recommends that a CM should be a nurse working at advanced practice level; district nurses are cited as being advanced practitioners with many inherent competencies in case management, assessment review, prescribing of medicines, supporting self-managed care, health promotion and prevention of ill health (DoH 2005a; NHS Modernisation Agency and Skills for Health, 2005e; DoH, 2005a,b). The CM will work with the patient to improve their medicines management using the performance criteria identified in the case management competences framework (NHS Modernisation Agency and Skills for Health, 2005). These include the following:

- monitoring and evaluating the use of medicines
- enabling patients to express their views and concerns

- discussing their needs and understanding of medicines, identifying and rectifying misconceptions
- enabling the patient to monitor their own reactions to medicines
- identifying newly acquired medicines and monitoring these for any changes in symptoms or health, maintaining an up-to-date list of medicines known to be used
- monitoring for possible side effects, multiple prescribing or any other problems
- identifying medicine risks and discussing these with patient
- identifying if medicines are taken as instructed, if not why?
- addressing non-compliance
- providing advice on where to get expert advice on medicines
- providing information about the medicines, effects of treatment, changes and combinations of prescriptions
- evaluating the administration of, storage, safety and disposal of medicines
- identifying the benefits and risks of compliance-informed decision making
- acting on concerns.

With proper support and advice and the identification of potential problems, CMs actively encourage patients to stay at home and function independently. Beasley (2005) highlights the need for CMs to:

- develop a personal care plan with the patient, carers, relatives and other health professionals based on a full assessment of their needs
- keep in touch and monitor the condition of the patient regularly, through home visits or telephone calls
- work in partnership with the patient's GP, sharing information and planning together.

A pilot study in Croydon is investigating the effectiveness of the 'virtual ward'. The CM will manage the virtual ward team which consists of nurses, a community pharmacist, social worker, physiotherapist, occupational therapist, administrator, voluntary sector representative and visiting physician or specialist nurses, and will work collaboratively with all disciplines involved in an individual's care. The virtual ward is a high dependency unit where high-risk patients are reviewed daily. This also includes a ward area where patients are reviewed weekly and an outpatients where expert patients and more stable patients are reviewed monthly, via virtual ward rounds and in virtual outpatients (Lewis, 2005).

Patient case study

The following example of interventions, actions and results highlights some common examples of how medication impacts on patient lives

Table 1.2 Case study Mr Ryan.

Intervention	Impact on patient	Result
Medication	Feels a bit better. Cancels GP appointment for review – does not want to waste valuable GP time	Inadequate glycaemic control unidentified. **Poor control of chronic condition**
Medication change	Requires insulin injections and is unable to self-administer. Dependent on nurse visiting at 9 am each morning, therefore has breakfast later than normal	Normal routine is disrupted and patient feels dependent
Monitoring method	Sore fingers. Stops playing piano at day centre, no purpose in going	Social isolation. Potential depression
Medication (anti-hypertensive) added at regular review	**Untolerated side effects affecting quality of life**, so patient stops taking them but does not tell GP. **Lack of concordance****	Increased risk of coronary heart disease and stroke
Repeat prescriptions	Each time insulin script is requested the patient also receives a supply of the initial anti-glycaemic and the anti-hypertensive	**Drug wastage**

*For explanation of the expert patient as defined by the DoH, see DOH (2004a, p. 15).
**For explanation of concordance as defined by the DoH, see DOH (2004a, p. 13).

Action for improvement	Outcome
Routine **regular review** at dedicated clinic identifying any problems with treatment, for example side effects, quality of life issues and effectiveness of treatment	Monitoring glycaemic control. Earlier identification of problems and earlier treatment interventions if required. **Reduction in hospital admissions**
Needs to learn how to self-administer insulin and have a wider knowledge base about his condition through education and information to restore independence. **Unmet need for high quality, evidence-based information about treatment**	With **education and support** he regains independence and preferred daily routine. Manages own condition effectively **The expert patient***
Utilise **evidence-based practice** (NICE, 2002). Reduce amount of glucose testing based on its effectiveness and giving the **patient** some **choice**, e.g. less frequent longer term blood monitoring	Patient's fingers recover and he returns to his normal social activity, thus resolving social isolation and resulting low mood
Professionals need to move away from the concept of compliance and work towards **concordance**	**Well informed** patients are better able to make treatment **choices** in **partnership** with appropriate professionals
Improving systems that generate repeat prescription to flag up regular review dates. Pharmacist support in identifying the return of unused prescribed drugs – **collaborative working**	GP alerted to drugs stopped by patient and **waste reduction**

Table 1.3 Case study – Mr. Ryan, part 2.

Intervention	Impact on patient	Result	Action for improvement	Result
Admitted to hospital as emergency via 999 call by neighbour after collapsing at home	No preparation; did not take own medication into hospital	Hospital staff unaware of current medication	Drug information cards. **Access to electronic patient records** (DoH, 2004c)	Hospital staff have record of current medication
Medication prescribed to control hypertension	Blood pressure reduced, patient feels well	Discharged on new tablets, continues to take old ones as well as no one knew he was on anything except insulin (reported by neighbour)	**Pre-discharge medication review. Explanation of changes to patient and carers and rationale for change**	Avoiding inappropriate over-medication
Patient takes discharge letter in sealed envelope to GP surgery; to save another journey he orders some more 'blood pressure tablets'	He has done as instructed and is unaware that the GP letter does not state the changed medication	He is prescribed his old 'blood pressure tablets', which were not effective	**Medication included on discharge letter. Ensure discharge letters are reviewed before any further changes made or prescriptions dispensed** (Randles & Black, 1999). **Electronic prescribing (NHS, 2006)**	Accurate and up-to-date prescribing
Patient takes prescription to pharmacist	Pharmacist dispenses 'old blood pressure tablets' from repeat prescription	Patient takes them instead of the new ones	**Discharge letter including medication copied to patient's preferred pharmacist** (Duggan et al., 1998)	Accurate and up-to-date dispensing

and how the experience may be improved with reference to the key areas (in bold) for improvement according to the medicines management resource document (DoH, 2004a), which are also supported by the other government documents previously mentioned.

Mr Ryan is a 75-year-old, independent gentleman who has a lot of respect for professionals and would not dream of questioning a decision or action on their part. He has been diagnosed as a type 2 diabetic and has been commenced on medication. The scenario shown in Table 1.2 ensues.

Summary of case study

The author suggests that the cornerstone to improvement in medicines management is good communication in terms of access, information, partnership, collaboration, choice and concordance. The DoH (2004a) supports this in discussion of joined up care between the primary and secondary sectors of health care. It is currently not uncommon for treatment to change in hospital and the patient is required to see the GP for further supplies. Several problems may arise at this point; see Table 1.3, using Mr Ryan again as an example.

Conclusion

Good management of medicines in older people involves a multi-disciplinary, collaborative approach that is co-ordinated by one key person who may be a CM or a community pharmacist. Everyone concerned, including the patient and carers, needs access to current information about the patient and their treatments. Every participant in the patient's care must endorse an excellent communication system in order to achieve good management and reduce risks. Patients and their carers need to have choices and remain central to any decision-making about their treatment and care in order to achieve concordance.

Implications for practice

Health professionals must enable the patient to be central to his/her own care decisions, providing one key care co-ordinator (case manager) who the patient can trust, rely on and discuss problems with; this may be the CM. The patient must be well informed in order to make choices and aid concordance.

Continued

All members of the multi-disciplinary team must share and learn from examples of good practice, learning from each other's mistakes and utilising technology to reduce risks of mistakes in prescribing, dispensing and administration of medicines. Improvements in channels of communication across the multi-disciplinary team assist the attainment of effective collaborative working, thus ensuring high quality care and support for the patients and their families.

The physiology of human ageing

2

Andy Evenden and Karen Gesty

Learning objectives

After completing this chapter, the reader will be able to:

- explain that physiological changes during normal human ageing occur as a result of alterations taking place at all levels of biological organisation
- appreciate that some ageing changes are clinically significant but other changes do not necessarily impact on normal physiology
- recognise that key ageing effects in the cardiovascular system occur largely as a result of the reduction in small vessel density, elastic vessel stiffening and myocardial cell loss/changes
- examine how a reduction in liver mass and a fall in hepatic blood flow with age can affect the metabolism (and bioavailability) of certain drugs
- explain how a fall in glomerular filtration rates and a reduced ability to control fluid and electrolyte balance can affect physiology and renal excretion of certain drugs
- identify that older people typically have a healthy immune system but it is different to that found in younger individuals and may have enhanced pro-inflammatory responses
- recognise that normal ageing effects of many body systems are typically masked by homeostatic compensatory processes, so problems may only occur when these mechanisms are exposed to additional stressors (such as exercise, ill-health or polypharmacy).

Introduction

The global rise in the population of older people has significant implications for health care. It could be argued, therefore, that the most important aspect of this phenomenon is an understanding by health care professionals of the physiological changes brought about during human ageing. Theories of human ageing and the history of scientific study into the ageing process make interesting reading but are sadly beyond the scope of this chapter. However, the authors would like to suggest some excellent sources where the interested reader may start their general studies into gerontology (see Kirkwood, 1999; Clark, 1999). In this chapter, we will limit our focus to a brief introduction regarding the concept of integrated human physiology before discussing the scale of biological changes that underpin the ageing process. This will include an insight into known age-related changes to key body organs and systems, as well as implications for practice.

Studies of human physiology in the twenty-first century, and the relationship between body processes and altered health states, mostly rely on a knowledge base of ever-increasing complexity. Recent advances in cellular and molecular biology have offered an insight into the intricate workings of the human body, but at the same time often present the reader with an impenetrable mass of scientific literature. An understanding of modern human physiology requires a set of unifying concepts and this can be provided by an appreciation of how body homeostasis is linked to the integrated action of biological processes at a number of organisation levels. The authors of this chapter presently employ this concept in their teaching of health care professionals across all academic levels and find it a robust model to explore human physiology and pathology issues.

Homeostasis and ageing

Homeostasis is the process of stabilising the internal environment of the body. In real terms, this is the use of complex physiological mechanisms to:

- maintain the composition of extracellular fluids
- provide the optimum conditions required for the normal operation of body cells.

Cells are the fundamental unit of the body, using many thousands of molecular interactions to carry out both basic and specialised functions. In turn, cells comprise the body's specific tissues, and tissues comprise the body's specific organs arranged into systems to maintain homeostasis. Consequently, we have a cyclical relationship, where cells maintain the homeostatic state that is essential for the survival of those same cells (see Figure 2.1a).

There are many theories about the nature of the mechanisms that underpin the ageing process in humans and other animals (see Kirkwood, 1999; Clark, 1999). It has been argued that ageing occurs as a result of inbuilt or 'programmed' genetic mechanisms (age-related changes), whilst it may also be the cumulative result of a life-time's

a)

b)

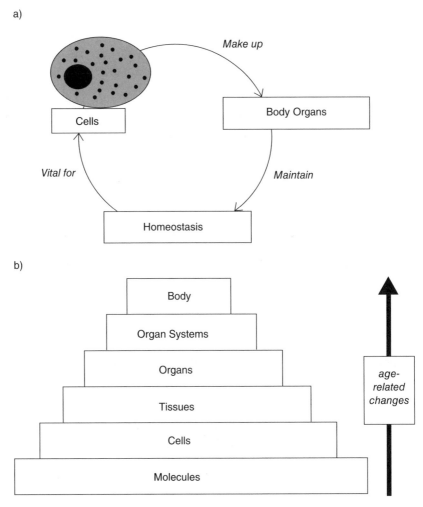

Figure 2.1 Human physiology and the ageing process (a) Human body systems exist to maintain homeostasis, which in turn is critical for cell function. (b) The relationship between molecular changes and the ageing process is such that small alterations in molecular aspects of cell function are expressed through changes to cells, tissues, organs and systems and ultimately body function.

wear and tear on a range of body systems (age-associated changes). Regardless of which theory is correct, it is increasingly evident that molecular and cellular changes are at the centre of any alteration, just like any normal human biological process (see Figure 2.1b).

The net effect of these changes has been effectively described by Rodwell et al. (2004) who noted (p. 2197):

> 'Functional decline in old age is not the result of the complete failure of a small number of cellular processes. Rather it is the slight weakening of many pathways that cumulatively causes a significant decrease in cell function.'

Consequently, to illustrate this point, this chapter will highlight those changes that occur to the cardiovascular system, the liver, the kidney and the immune system, with particular implications for medication management.

Prior to our review of physiological changes in ageing, the authors would like to bring to the reader's attention a few key facts. Many studies into the physiology of older people are based on extrapolations of research findings from laboratory animals and/or sometimes arbitrarily selected populations that fail to reflect health status or any defined age category. In addition, readers will be aware of the National Service Framework for Older People, where three age classes are used; entering old age (50+ and largely socially constructed), transitional phase (normally 70+ and becoming frail) and frail older people (DoH 2001a). The majority of the research in the following review will not specifically address these individual classes. However, we have endeavoured where possible to highlight the relevance of research findings to health care practice and, more pertinently, to medication management.

Ageing and the cardiovascular system

The cardiovascular system, consisting of the heart and vascular tree, is vital for fluid and molecule transport needed to maintain the millions of body cells. Therefore, any reduction in function regarding the individual components of this system has potentially severe effects. Physiological ageing in the cardiovascular system assumes many forms, with cardiovascular dysfunction remaining a significant cause of mortality and morbidity in the elderly. Changes to cardiovascular physiology should be a major consideration in any physical examination, diagnostic process or treatment regime involving the older person. A number of normal ageing events are recognised in the cardiovascular system, as well as disease-related changes facilitated by conditions including atherosclerosis and hypertensive cardiovascular disease

(Taffet & Lakatta, 1999). Normal and pathological ageing processes can be highly variable in their presentation and development. In addition, they may be significantly influenced by lifestyle factors where diet, smoking and exercise levels impact on the health of the older person. An overview of age-related and age-associated changes to the cardio-vascular system can be seen in Figure 2.2.

Changes to the vascular system

The vascular tree will be considered as a separate organ for the purpose of this chapter. It is affected by a number of distinct age-associated structural and functional changes, including incremental stiffening and elongation of the large elastic arteries. The body's gradual response to these changes is a net increase in the diameter of the arterial lumen which, when measured at the aortic root, can increase in size up to 20% over the period between 30 years and 80 years of age. This change is thought to compensate for arterial stiffening by permitting a decrease in pulse pressure. However, the increased volume of blood that needs to be moved during systole can increase the overall work of the heart (Lakatta & Sollot, 2002).

Smaller arteries appear to be less affected by structural changes, as the wall thickness and luminal diameters tend to increase with age but with no associated change in vessel distensibility (Lakatta & Sollot, 2002). Possibly the most significant change to smaller arteries is a reduction in the formation of new vessels (angiogenesis) after isch-aemic trauma. This has serious implications for the remodelling of vital cerebral and coronary arteries after pathological insult. The capillary bed is also subject to change with advancing age; whilst new vessel formation would appear to occur as normal, there is a general decrease in the number and density of capillaries in many organs. These capil-lary changes are of particular relevance to the administration of drugs, as the reduced tissue perfusion (compounded by a decrease in tissue mass and body water content) affects the dissemination and distribu-tion of medication. For example, intra-muscular injections are likely to take longer to exert their pharmacological effects in older people, due to these cumulative changes.

Little research has been carried out regarding the effects of age on the body's veins. However, the common femoral vein experiences a decline in diameter and associated blood velocity, which affects the flow of blood to the leg. The capacitance of veins for blood is seen to decrease in older people, and individuals may also have venous func-tion impaired via valvular insufficiency and varicosities (Taffet & Lakatta, 1999). Such venous insufficiency in the older person contrib-utes, along with both individual genetic and lifestyle factors, to the development of conditions such as oedema, phlebitis and chronic leg ulceration.

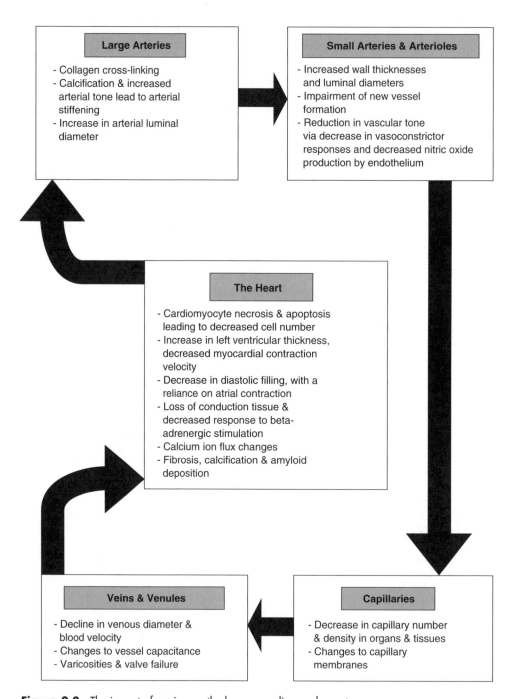

Figure 2.2 The impact of ageing on the human cardiovascular system.

Changes to cardiac tissue

The heart is affected by a variety of structural and functional changes with increasing age (Kitzman & Edwards, 1990). Post-mortem examinations provide evidence that an increased cardiac mass occurs, particularly in older women. Specifically, there is an increase in the thickness of the left ventricular wall, which may expand by up to 50% between a person's third and ninth decade. The aged heart is also found to be more fibrotic, with a patchy network of collagen between cells. Calcification and additional fibrotic changes may also be present in the cardiac valves and septum. Innervation of the heart appears to change during ageing, with a reduction in both parasympathetic and sympathetic neurones, affecting the electrical conduction pathways that drive myocardial contractions. In many individuals there is deposition of cardiac amyloid protein, typically in the atria. Amyloid is the name given to a fibrous extracellular insoluble protein aggregate, formed by (age-associated) mutation to the genes encoding specific proteins. It is a common feature of ageing in many tissues, including the brain. Amyloid deposition in the atrium may interfere with the conduction of electrical impulses important for muscular contraction and therefore may contribute to the increased tendency in older persons to develop atrial fibrillation. Amyloid deposits in the endothelium of the heart (and other tissues and organs) may also act as a stimulus for inappropriate blood clotting and explain some thrombotic events in older people.

Changes to cardiovascular function and control

Many changes to heart function are associated with diastolic competency rather than systolic effects, resulting in no significant clinical changes to cardiac output, ventricular ejection fraction or the resting heart rate. However, there is a marked fall regarding early diastolic filling of the left ventricle caused by impaired relaxation (Kitzman et al., 2002). Older people have an increased reliance on left atrial contractions to compensate for this fault in relaxation and in 80 year olds there may be up to a 40% reliance on this compensation effect, compared with 10% in youth. This may explain why atrial fibrillation events are less well tolerated in older people and why cardiac output may be less adaptable after exercise.

There are no serious changes to the overall heart rate in the elderly, although there are marked changes to the intrinsic heart rate (the basic rate without external controlling nervous and hormonal influences). Parasympathetic nervous control is diminished compared with the control of heart rate seen in the young, reflected by a reduced effect of atropine on the aged heart rate. The variability of heart rate is also seen to decrease with age, with the lowest and highest daily heart rates being lower than that of a younger person. This is probably a result of changes to the sinoatrial node and other tissues of the electrical conduction system. ECG recordings show gradual alterations, with the PR interval lengthening with age. The upper limits are 220 ms in those over the age of 65, compared with a mean time of 200 ms in younger people. Other ECG changes can be a flattening of the ST segment and T waves with a smaller magnitude. Changes to the ST segment and T waves can also be caused by a range of medications such as digoxin, diuretics, antiarrhythmics or psychoactive drugs. These changes to the ECG in the absence of co-presenting pathologies are mainly benign, and probably reflect subtle effects of past insults and changes to cells and tissues highlighted below. In fact, in the very old (100+), many ECG abnormalities have been noted and it is very rare to find an entirely normal trace in this age group.

There is evidence to suggest that the baroreceptor reflex (an important mechanism for blood pressure homeostasis) is altered during ageing. One manifestation of the decreased responsiveness of this reflex is the occurrence of orthostatic hypotension, (the fall in blood pressure observed when an upright posture is adopted). The decrease in heart rate seen after an acute rise in blood pressure is lower in older people than in younger subjects. In addition, the increase in heart rate after a fall in blood pressure is less pronounced. It is not known whether this effect is a function of changes to the heart (as the effector organ), or as a result of defects in the vascular receptor tissue. It is clear that the hearts of older people exhibit a reduced capacity for compensation, but this is often less important in a clinical context than the existence of specific pathologies and/or the physical activity status of a patient.

Key changes to cardiovascular tissues involve alterations to both cardiac and smooth muscle and the extracellular matrix. The characteristic stiffening of arterial walls can be attributed to fragmentation of elastin fibres and an increase in collagen content, with (glucose-mediated) cross linking of collagen in the sub-endothelium of the vessel. Such collagen changes are found in many cardiovascular tissues during ageing but are particularly increased in the arterial tunica media. There is also some evidence of a similar collagen effect in capillary walls. The collagen subtypes found in cardiovascular tissues may also undergo change. A particular form (type I filaments) increases in number and thickness in the heart of older people, resulting in increased stiffening of the tissue. Calcification is another feature of these age-associated changes, where calcium salts deposited in the tissues of the heart and large arteries also result in stiffening effects.

Changes to cardiovascular cells

Cellular changes are evident throughout the cardiovascular system with advancing age. In the elastic arteries, endothelial cells undergo enlargement and appear to have an irregularity in size, shape and contour. There is also a hypertrophic increase in smooth muscle cells. Alterations to the left ventricular wall are in part due to the loss of the cardiac muscle cells (cardiomyocytes), with the remaining cells undergoing morphological changes to increase cell length and cross-sectional area. This 'drop-out' of myocytes and other cells in the cardiovascular system is thought to occur by one of two major cell-death mechanisms. One mechanism results in cell death over time as a result of post-traumatic (or post-toxic) necrosis. Alternatively, cells may be lost via programmed cell death or apoptosis (Husse et al., 2003). Apoptosis is a key process in tissue remodelling and may be stimulated by a range of insults, although the exact mechanism remains unclear. The function of cardiac muscle cells is also affected by modifications to the flux of calcium ions in older cells. The resting stores of calcium in the myocytes appear to decrease with advancing age and additionally, the amount of calcium taken up by cell storage compartments is less than in the young heart. As a result of these changes, cardiac muscle cell contraction can be slower. The shortest time interval between cardiomyocyte contractions in the old heart is considerably longer than in young myocardial tissue.

Other significant cellular changes in the vascular system relate to the ability of cells to respond to extracellular signals, affecting both receptor sensitivity and signal transduction. For example, α-adrenergic responses associated with vasoconstriction are relatively conserved, but β-adrenergic responses associated with vasodilation are found to decrease with age (Bressler & Bahl, 2003). In addition, changes to signalling mechanisms (important in vascular control) occur with a fall in the responsiveness of the renin-angiotensin system and a decrease in nitric oxide-mediated vasodilation. These changes mean that older people typically have less control over the constriction and dilation of their blood vessels.

Implications for practice

Changes to cardiovascular physiology are often masked and compounded by accompanying pathologies, such as atherosclerotic and ischaemic disease, and healthy function is strongly influenced by lifestyle factors such as levels of physical activity. Vascular changes with age include a tendency for the smaller arteries to become less able to remodel themselves after trauma and insult, with decreases in capillary densities in tissues and organs and an increase in venous insufficiency through valvular defects and varicosities. Therefore, vascular ageing can have a significant effect on wound healing, tissue fluid levels and the efficacy of drug administration via decreases in tissue perfusion.

Continued

Cardiac function is also affected by age and, apart from the well-characterised effects of common cardiac pathologies (such as ischaemic trauma), the heart can demonstrate a reduced capacity for physiological compensation, particularly during and after exercise.

Hepatic ageing

The human liver is one of the body's most important organs, performing a vast array of metabolic and regulatory processes. Its key functions are:

- bile production
- biotransformation of drugs and other substances
- plasma protein production, e.g. albumin, prothrombin
- nutrient processing, e.g. deamination of amino-acids
- removal of old blood cells by Kupffer cell phagocytosis
- storage, e.g. iron, glycogen.

Schmucker (2001) noted that 'the most remarkable characteristic of liver function in the elderly is the increase in inter-individual variability, a feature that may obscure age-related differences' (p. 837). The healthy liver has a large functional reserve and clinical studies provide little evidence to indicate a reduction in hepatic performance with age. However, healthy individuals do show a reduction in liver size, blood flow and perfusion by approximately 35% between the third and tenth decade (Hall, 2003). Hepatic blood supply tends to fall with age, largely as a result of gradual decreases to cardiac output and a reduction in the blood flow supplying the abdominal viscera (splanchnic flow). Total hepatic mass is tightly regulated throughout life and the liver continues to possess the ability to grow or shrink relatively quickly in order to meet metabolic demands even in the over-65s, e.g. following injury or transplant. In humans, the liver normally comprises approximately 2.5% total body weight until approximately 70 years but this may decline to around 1.6% after 90 years (Mezey, 2003).

Changes to hepatic tissue

Two-thirds of the liver is made of parenchyma and the remainder is the biliary tract. Parenchyma comprises functional hepatocytes, which are responsible for the liver's metabolic actions. Parenchyma may undergo fibrosis and gradual loss of function with advancing age, but this does not indicate cirrhosis. The body can tolerate up to three-quarters of the parenchyma being damaged before liver function is compromised as a result of hepatocyte loss. There is a reduction in hepatic volume by approximately 17–28% between the ages of 40 and 65 (Merck, 2005), and the linear relationship between liver weight and body surface area also decreases with age. It is believed that this reduction in liver size has an impact on drug clearance rates. An ageing liver is browner than its younger counterparts, thought to be due to an accumulation of lipofuscin pigment (cross-linked protein and lipid residues, formed by age-associated oxidative processes) in hepatocytes. However, it is not known if this finding is of clinical significance at present.

Changes to hepatic cells

Histological changes have been detected in the ageing liver, which may signal degenerative hepatic processes (such as hepatocyte loss) or, alternatively, the operation of compensatory mechanisms (such as changes to mitochondria structures). However, the clinical significance of these cellular changes is currently unclear. Giant hepatocytes are more prevalent and an increase in nuclear size has been noted; the nucleus may also contain more than the diploid number of chromosomes (Timiras, 2002). In addition, the number of mitochondria per hepatocyte typically decreases with age (although there may be an increase in mitochondrial size) and a fall in the amount of endoplasmic reticulum occurs. An increase in the number of hepatic lysosomes has also been observed. Unlike some body cells, hepatocytes are known to regenerate throughout life although their rate of turnover decreases with advancing age, possibly due to a reduced ability to respond to growth factors (Schmucker, 1998).

The liver has a highly specialised capillary bed, to facilitate the transfer of substrates from the blood to the hepatocytes. Normally, the capillary walls (sinusoidal endothelium) have many fenestrations or pores, with no basal lamina – leading some researchers to refer to them as the 'liver sieve'. However, electron microscopy studies have highlighted a significant age-related thickening of the liver sinusoidal endothelium (termed pseudocapillarisation), causing a loss of fenestrations and new basal lamina formation (McLean et al., 2003). Defenestration of this endothelium is associated with a reduced hepatic ability to remove plasma lipids, and Hilmer et al. (2005) proposed that this inability to remove lipoproteins provided a mechanism for linking ageing changes to the disease process atherosclerosis (see Figure 2.3).

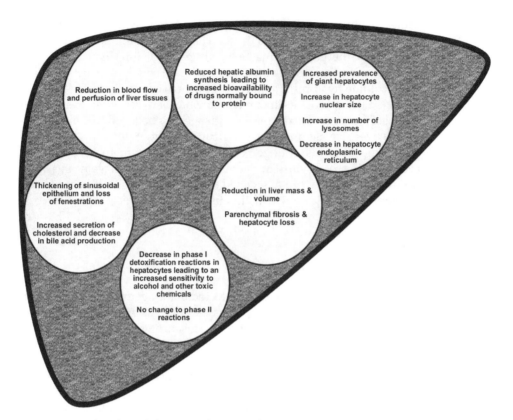

Figure 2.3 Physiological changes to the ageing liver.

Changes to hepatic molecular biology

Serum and biliary cholesterol levels appear to rise with increasing age
(Schmucker, 1998). This is thought to be a result of enhanced hepatic
secretion of cholesterol (including enhanced intestinal absorption) and
decreased bile acid synthesis and secretion. In addition, the gallbladder
appears to have a reduced sensitivity to the intestinal hormone chole-
cystokinin with age, causing it to have sluggish contractions and permitting bile sludge to be retained for a longer period of time. This may
explain why advancing age is a known risk factor for development of
cholesterol gallstones.

The liver plays an important role in pharmacokinetics and the metabolic breakdown and removal of a drug by the liver is known as the
first pass mechanism. These biotransformation activities are largely
carried out by two main processes, termed Phase 1 and Phase 2 reactions, which break down molecules (drugs) into water-soluble metabolites ready for excretion. Phase 1 reactions are typically performed by

hepatic enzymes (from the cytochrome p450 system) and comprise oxidation, reduction and hydrolysis. These reactions occur inside the endoplasmic reticulum of hepatocytes and are known to gradually decrease with age. However, the decrease in Phase 1 reactions is considered to be an effect of a reduced liver mass and hepatic blood flow rather than a failing of the enzymes themselves (Schmucker, 2001). Phase 1 reactions are responsible for the breakdown of drugs such as alcohol. Consequently, a reduction in these processes contributes to making older people more prone to the effects of alcohol, e.g. drowsiness, when compared with younger individuals consuming a similar amount. Phase 2 reactions largely occur in the cytosol and result in the conjugation of drugs with a polar molecule, such as cysteine, glycine or glutathione to facilitate renal excretion. Phase 2 reactions are responsible for clearing drugs such as temazepam and valproic acid. These reactions appear to remain unchanged with age, possibly due to additional extrahepatic (e.g. intestinal mucosa, lung, kidney) conjugation activity.

After absorption, a large number of drugs bind to plasma proteins produced by the liver, which inactivates the compound until it is released. The rest of the unbound fraction of the drug is responsible for its effects in the body. One of the main plasma proteins responsible for this binding action is albumin, but its hepatic production appears to fall with increasing age (Livingstone, 2003). Whilst this fall is not usually clinically significant by itself, it can result in an increased bioavailability of certain drugs which are normally tightly bound to plasma proteins (such as warfarin), particularly if there are other pathologies present, e.g. renal or liver disease, or in situations of polypharmacy (when other drugs may compete for the same binding proteins). It is advisable to prescribe drugs that are bound in this way in low doses and to increase their amounts slowly.

Implications for practice

A range of age-related changes are seen in the liver, but liver function is well preserved in the healthy older person. There is no single standardised test to assess hepatic function. As liver function becomes increasingly variable between individuals as they age, the effects on drug clearance become harder to assess, particularly in the presence of polypharmacy and accompanying pathologies. The aphorism of 'start low, go slow' when prescribing drugs to older patients would appear to reflect some of the hepatic changes particularly concerning Phase 1 reactions and plasma proteins, which are more likely to be reduced in older individuals.

Renal ageing

An age-related decline in human kidney function is evident from laboratory tests after the relatively early age of 30, and by the age of 85 years renal function has been reduced by half, although there is great variation regarding age of onset, nature and speed of renal deterioration (Timiras & Leary, 2002). Renal degenerative effects are typically slow to develop, and display both structural and physiological features. The term renal senescence has been used to encompass changes at the organ, tissue, cellular and molecular level (Melk & Halloran, 2001).

A reduction in renal weight of 25% has been reported with increasing age, with ultrasound studies showing a loss of approximately 15% in length between the ages of 30 and 85 years (Miletic et al., 1998). As a person ages, the amount of parenchymal tissue in the kidney is progressively reduced, particularly in the cortex region. This atrophy results in a smaller organ but one that is still effective. However, a decrease in overall efficiency often occurs when older kidneys are under an increased workload (such as stress, illness and medications). In addition, a gradual reduction in renal blood flow occurs with increasing age that may also be exacerbated by pathological effects such as hypertension, which can compromise glomerular vasculature.

Changes to tubular function

The best overall index of kidney function is taken to be the glomerular filtration rate (GFR). This can be clinically calculated in a number of ways but perhaps the most commonly encountered method is by measuring creatinine (a metabolite of muscle tissue) in a timed urine sample. The production and excretion of creatinine both decline with age, due to a concomitant decrease in lean (muscle) tissue and a reduced GFR. As a urine sample may be difficult to obtain in older people, a simpler method to determine creatinine clearance is often used known as the Cockcroft-Gault approximation. This assumes a renal function decrease of 1 ml/min/year after the age of 40. However, approximately 30% of the population show no fall in GFR with age (Wiggins, 2003), and Luke & Beck (1999) note that this is not a well authenticated method for assessing individuals above 70 years of age.

In approximately 70% of the population, the ageing kidney can be characterised by a reduced GFR, with a loss of nephrons and a narrowed homeostatic ability to control water and electrolyte balance (Wiggins, 2003). This means there is less surface area available for filtration, and the glomerular membrane may become more permeable. As renal tubular function decreases, a reduction in urinary concentrating ability (particularly in individuals over 65) has an increasing impact on body fluid balance. These older individuals typically experience a decreased sensation of thirst in response to dehydration, making them more susceptible to life-threatening variations in hyperosmolality and hypovolemia (Tian et al., 2004). It has also been noted that adults over 65 subsequently drink less water following periods of exercise in a warm environment and so suffer a delay in full restoration of fluid balance (Kenney & Chiu, 2001).

Total urine output does not significantly change with increasing age, but the diurnal rhythm becomes altered, possibly due to variations in vasopressin secretion (Asplund et al., 1998). This typically has the effect of causing older people (over 60) to produce urine at a similar rate in both day and night time, so increasing nocturia, unlike younger people who usually produce more urine in the day. Attempts by older people to reduce the impact of this annoyance commonly involve individuals reducing their fluid intake during the evenings; however, this could exacerbate a precarious fluid balance.

A reduction in the number and size of kidney nephrons with age (evident after the fourth decade of life) could eventually lead to pharmacological complications. This may particularly involve the accumulation of drugs whose removal is reliant partly (or totally) on renal excretion of the intact form, e.g. digoxin, cimetidine, lithium and many antimicrobial agents (Rehman, 2004). However, McLean & LeCouteur (2004) found that renal drug clearance and glomerular filtration rate are reduced in older people with underlying renal disease, but are typically well preserved and effective in many healthy older people; so renal complications and old age are not necessarily synonymous.

Cellular ageing in the kidney is generally characterised by a thickening of the glomerular basement membrane, accompanied by localised (focal) glomerulosclerosis and mesangial cell expansion (Wiggins, 2003). These changes are thought to affect the ability to process urine. Cells in the kidney replicate at a slow rate and some cells, e.g. podocytes, do not replicate at all (termed 'post-mitotic'), which makes repair difficult. Podocytes are specialised epithelial cells that comprise the main part of the glomerular filtration barrier in the kidney. Age-associated damage and subsequent loss of podocytes appears to result in exposed areas of basement membrane in some glomeruli. This is thought to be the trigger for the sclerosing process, which involves segments of the glomerulus losing vital cell structures, with normal features being replaced by extracellular matrix. Eventually the whole glomerulus may be affected and so degenerate, resulting in a scattering of scarred nephron structures and interstitial fibrosis in the renal cortex, reducing filtration rate and efficiency.

Mesangial cells are a type of smooth muscle cell, located around blood capillaries in the glomerulus. They are able to contract and so play a regulatory role by affecting the blood flow through the glomerulus. Mesangial cells also contribute to extracellular matrix production in the kidney and secrete a variety of other vasoactive substances, including prostaglandins. The observed increase in mesangial cell number is thought to be an age-related benign feature, rather than a pathological one.

A functional genomics approach has identified 958 genes in the human kidney that change expression with age. However, to date, no specific genes are known to be clinically significant with regards to effects such as age-related glomerulosclerosis. Extracellular proteins may react with sugars under oxidative conditions in the human body and form advanced glycation end products (AGEs). The altered release of growth factors and cytokines in the ageing kidney reflects accumulation of AGEs in renal tissues and in addition, lipofuscin pigment is known to accumulate in aged podocytes. However, it is not known if these changes are a direct cause or effect of ageing, or whether they have a significant function in a clinical context. Locally produced vasodilatory prostaglandins and nitric oxide (NO) play an important role in the maintenance of healthy renal perfusion. Consequently, ageing changes in the cardiovascular system involving falling NO levels, and alterations in vascular tone can also reduce the kidney's ability to filter and process urine effectively with age.

Implications for practice

The kidney experiences significant age-related changes, which are clinically measurable, typically resulting in a fall in the glomerular filtration rate and a reduction in tubular function. This has clinical significance as it may lead to an accumulation in the blood of those drugs that are actively secreted by the kidney, causing toxicity.

Ageing and the immune system

An examination of the major diseases associated with human ageing reveals a number of pathologies relatively rare in younger individuals with optimally functioning immune systems. The common causes of morbidity and mortality in older people include bacterial and viral infections, and autoimmune and inflammatory pathologies (such as diabetes and arthritis), as well as an increase in benign and malignant tumours. Such life-limiting disorders have provided the main impetus for the study of the ageing process on the immune system, a phenomenon termed immunosenescence. Immunosenescence is linked to changes in a number of immune parameters, reflecting alterations at the level of organs, tissues, cells and molecules (Franceschi et al., 2000).

Changes to organs and tissues

The major structures of the immune system are the organs of the thymus and spleen and the disseminated tissues that comprise bone marrow, lymph nodes and mucosal associated lymphoid tissues (such as Peyer's patches in the intestinal tract). One of the most notable age-related changes in the immune tissues is found in the thymus gland. This organ experiences a reduction in size throughout adult life, becoming less organised in structure and losing a significant proportion of its component cells. Such changes in organ morphology are followed by changes in biochemical and physiological functions, notably a reduction in the export of T-lymphocytes and a reduction in variety of T-cell subtypes (Andrew & Aspinall, 2002). Another age-related immune tissue change involves bone marrow. A decrease in the developmental precursors to B-lymphocytes suggests changes to bone marrow stromal cells but the exact nature of these changes is unknown. The reduction in numbers and variability in both B and T-lymphocytes may be an important factor in the remodelling of the immune system in older persons.

Changes to immune cells

The immune system is a highly cellular entity and immune functions are largely reliant on the actions of discrete cell populations. These populations include macrophages, neutrophils and natural killer (NK) cells of innate (non-specific) immunity, as well as differentiated lymphocytes involved with adaptive (specific) immune functions. In non-specific immunity, cell functions can remain potent even in the oldest members of our society. However, there is evidence of reduced communication between antigen-presenting cells and T-lymphocytes, as well as a number of age-related changes regarding NK cells, which results in an impaired function in older people (Ginaldi & Sternberg, 2002), possibly affecting the ability to target tumours. B-lymphocytes exhibit a decline in their proliferative capacity, with a decrease in circulating cells and cell diversity. These changes may have some clinical significance for older persons, as the incidence of pathological conditions involving B-cells (such as the production of autoantibodies and B-cell leukaemias) increases with age. In addition, many changes to antibody levels could be explained by immune defects, such as reduced cytokine activities, as part of a declining and defective B-cell influence with age.

T-lymphocytes are central to the cell-mediated adaptive immune process and Pawelec et al. (2001) noted age-associated effects on the various T-cell subsets in the body. There is a general decline in T-cell production, with T-cells becoming less responsive and experiencing a change in the proportion of memory and activated T-cells, compared to the total population of naive T-cells. Naive T-cells also appear to have a reduced response during encounters with antigens. There is also evidence of an increase in senescent T-cells, due to faults in apoptosis which would normally remove these cells from the body's tissues. One theory regarding immunosenescence is that, as the body ages and is exposed to increasing antigenic challenges, the populations of memory cells increase until there is little 'immunological space' (Franceschi et al., 2000). Reduction in immunological space would clearly influence both the responsiveness and adaptability of the immune system and goes some way to explaining the changes in disease susceptibility seen in older people.

Changes to immune molecules

Some of the most profound changes to the immune system that accompany ageing occur at a molecular level. Changes in antibody production (humoral immunity) stimulated by changes to lymphocytes are also related to considerable alterations in the cytokine profile of older people (Gardener & Murasko, 2002). There is a marked increase in cytokines such as Interleukin 1 (IL1), Interleukin 6 (IL6) and Tumour Necrosis Factor (TNFα) molecules. These are regarded as pro-inflammatory signals and are produced by mononuclear immune cells. These changes may explain some of the pathological alterations in ageing individuals, such as rheumatoid arthritis, osteoporosis and atherosclerosis. In general, age-related changes to cytokine production promote a skewing of the immunological response away from a balance between cell-mediated (Th1) and humoral reactions (Th2), to a predominance of Th2 reactions. This shift in balance may explain the increased rate of infections, the increase in neoplastic growth and reactivation of latent viral infections often seen in older persons.

Ageing and the inflammatory response

The tendency of older people to develop a more inflammation-oriented immune system is connected with a spectrum of presenting conditions found with increasing age. Inflammation involves a complex series of cellular and molecular interactions, which enable an individual to respond quickly to tissue trauma and infection. This process involves the prevention of microorganism dissemination, their ultimate destruction and the successful repair and healing of affected tissues (Nathan,

2002). The influence of inflammation on the well-being of older people ranges from the general increase in 'aches and pains' through to delayed wound healing and to chronic inflammatory pathologies. Conclusive proof of cause and effect with regard to increased inflammation in the older person and the increased incidence of certain pathologies is still hard to find. However, practitioners with regular contact with older people should be aware that inflammation is one of the most contemporary topics in biomedicine and future research findings are likely to have a significant impact on gerontology and geriatric medicine.

Implications for practice

The human immune system undergoes a remodelling with age rather than a decline in all its functions. The highly co-ordinated cellular adaptive immune responses appear to be those most affected by age, whilst pro-inflammatory responses may actually increase. The cellular deficits in the immune system may be precipitated by loss of thymus tissue, bone marrow senescence and a reduction in co-ordinating cytokine systems. Susceptibility to infection, auto-immune pathologies and tumour formation are not solely initiated by an immune dysfunction, and there is a possibility that a lack of immune responsiveness in older people occurs as a result of a lack of 'immunological space'. Inflammatory responses are responsible for a large number of commonly encountered chronic diseases in older people and phenomena such as delayed wound healing. The successful moderation of inflammatory pathways may have clinical benefit in the future.

Apart from the specific alteration to components of the immune response, health care practitioners should be aware of the influence of other key physiological parameters on the body's ability to defend itself. In practice, factors such as adequate nutrition, hydration and personal hygiene will play an important role in maintaining the body's various defences, and pathological changes (such as alterations to tissue blood flow and the presence of pulmonary disease) can all influence an individual's likelihood of acquiring an infection.

Implications for practice summary

Rehman (2004) highlighted that 'age-related changes in drug metabolism are a complicated interplay between genetics, ageing, disease and environment' (p. 24). Much is still to be discovered about the impact of age-related physiological changes on the pharmacological responses of older people, especially

Continued

as they are rarely recruited to drug trials or considered in reviews of efficacy. It is also possible that some of the physiological changes highlighted here may become increasingly relevant with the development of new medications. Consequently, practitioners are invited to consider the implications of ageing physiology outlined in this chapter with regards to both their current and possible future practice.

The application of applied pharmacology to the older person

Maggi Banning

Learning objectives

This chapter aims to provide the reader with an introduction to the principles of pharmacology, namely pharmacokinetics and pharmacodynamics. The chapter aims to achieve the following:

- an introduction to pharmacology with an examination of the processes of drug absorption, drug metabolism and drug excretion
- the impact of ageing on these pharmacokinetic parameters
- an explanation of the mode of action of drugs or pharmacodynamics
- an introduction to how drugs interact with receptors, ion channels, enzyme inhibiting sites or receptor operated ion channels
- an examination of the impact of ageing on pharmacodynamics and the need for pharmacovigilance.

Introduction

Pharmacology is the study of the effects of drugs and how they are used to treat medical conditions. This area of science may be separated into pharmacokinetics, which is the mathematical assessment of the influence of the body on the drug and can manifest itself in drug absorption, drug distribution, drug metabolism and drug excretion (O'Mahony, 2000); and pharmacodynamics, which refers to the mode

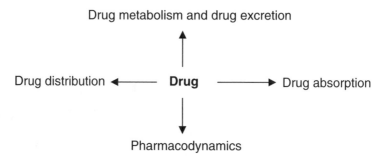

Figure 3.1   Pharmacological processes involved in the pathway of drugs.

of action of drugs or what the drug does to the body. To understand drug action and its role in the treatment of pathophysiological conditions, nurses caring for patients, nurse prescribers and community matrons need to comprehend both the pharmacokinetic and pharmacodynamics properties of drugs (see Figure 3.1). By doing this, nurses and prescribers will have a greater comprehension of the role of specific medicines in the management of selected conditions and will be able to recognise potential pharmacological toxicity.

Drug absorption

Drugs are administered in numerous ways. The route of administration will determine how quickly a drug is absorbed, for example a drug administered intravenously will have direct access to the blood stream, whereas a drug administered orally will have to pass the gastric or intestinal mucosa in order to be absorbed. The cell membrane is the first barrier which drugs meet in terms of absorption. Membranes are ubiquitous within the body and are composed of two layers of lipid (lipid bilayer), with pores that allow drugs to pass through by passive diffusion, filtration, facilitated diffusion or active transport.

The most common method of transport is passive diffusion. This involves the ability of the drug to pass through the lipid component of the membrane. The passive diffusion of drugs through cell membranes is dependent on three factors: lipid solubility, the concentration gradient across the membrane and the ionisation status of the drug.

The concentration gradient is a physical state of the plasma membrane and is generated by osmosis or the energy source that enables drugs to pass from the exterior to the interior of the cell. The rate of diffusion is proportional to the concentration gradient across the membrane. The ionisation status is the ability of the compound to dissociate into ions or charged particles when in solution. This property is a physicochemical state of each drug. For good absorption it is necessary for drugs to remain non-ionised. The gastrointestinal tract is lined with a plasma membrane, so drugs that are administered by either an oral or a rectal route can be transported by passive diffusion provided they possess these key characteristics.

Drugs can also be transported across the plasma membrane using a variety of mechanisms, including facilitated diffusion, active transport or carrier mediated transport. Because of the physicochemical nature of many drugs, they are unable to pass through the plasma membrane unhindered. In these cases, drugs employ the use of a carrier molecule or protein embedded within the plasma membrane to assist their transport across the membrane. Drugs that are transported in this way are also regulated by their molecular weight, physicochemical properties, the thickness of the plasma membrane and the flow of water across the membrane. For example, water-soluble drugs such as aspirin may either by transported using aqueous channels or use a carrier protein to aid their transport through the pores of the membrane. However, not all body tissues possess a lipid bilayer. The lungs have a large surface area but possess only a single membrane that is permeable to lipid soluble and insoluble drugs; for example, drugs in the form of toxic gases, volatile solvents and aerosols rapidly pass across the membrane surface to be transported to the alveoli of the lungs. This rapid blood flow through the alveolar spaces and interstitial spaces allows the quick uptake of many volatile and lipid soluble drugs by passive diffusion.

Factors that alter the absorption of drugs

Drug absorption may be altered due to changes in gastric emptying time, pH of the intestinal tract, active transport within the gut or blood flow (Bender, 1968). In older people, the gastrointestinal tract is subjected to age-related changes which may involve reduced gastrointestinal blood flow, atrophy of gastric and intestinal mucosa and decline in splanchic perfusion; both may marginally reduce drug absorption (Dharmarajan & Ugalino, 2001; Hämmerlein et al., 1998). The older person may also have slightly elevated gastric pH which can affect the transit of certain drugs; for example, the intragastric metabolism of levodopa may be impaired leading to a reduction of dopa decarboxylase and a three-fold increase in the availability of levodopa (Evans et al., 1980).

Often drugs can be metabolised within the liver following oral absorption and then excreted immediately before being circulated to the systemic circulation. This is referred to as the 'first-pass' effect (or pre-systemic elimination); this can increase the bioavailability of drugs (Peck, 1985; Lamy, 1990). In the older person, the first-pass effect through the liver is reduced. Older people may also exhibit reduced absorption of antibiotics at intramuscular injection sites (Douglas et al.,

1980); this can cause problems when treating infection with antimicro-bials (Hammerlein et al., 1998). Following absorption, drugs are dis-tributed to the cardiovascular system and from there are transported to other organ systems such as the lungs, brain and liver.

Drug distribution

After drugs have been absorbed, they are distributed to the plasma where the drug will bind to the plasma proteins albumin or α_1-glyco-protein. Protein binding is a hypothetical physiological mechanism that aims to maintain equilibrium between the amount of drug that is maintained in the serum which is inactive (protein bound) and the amount that is not bound to protein and therefore free to cross plasma membranes and exert a biological effect. As the free drug is metabo-lised, the concentration of free drug falls, which is the trigger for the release of an equivalent amount of drug from the protein bound fraction. Eventually the total concentration of drug will be exhausted as the serum levels reduce to zero. The physicochemical properties of each drug specify the extent of protein binding, for example, aspirin is 50% bound and 50% free.

Protein binding can be viewed as a safety measure which aims to reg-ulate the amount of drug that is free to exert a biological effect, and at the same time maintain the serum levels within a therapeutic level. The binding of drugs to albumin can be affected by polypharmacy. Drugs with different binding affinities compete for binding sites on albumin; when several drugs compete for binding sites, some drugs can be com-petitively displaced rendering them unbound and therefore free to exert a biological effect. A common example is that of warfarin and the use of non-steroidal anti-inflammatory drugs (NSAIDs) such as voltarol. Voltarol possesses a lower plasma protein binding capacity and occupies about 50% of the binding sites at therapeutic concentrations (Rang et al., 2000), and therefore displaces warfarin from its binding sites allowing more free or unbound drug to exert its biological effect. This displace-ment reaction can increase the risk of dose-dependent bleeding.

In the older person, drug distribution is affected in several ways. The most important effects include an increase in body fat by as much as 15–30% and reductions in lean body mass and total body water (Forbes & Reina, 1970). These changes can lead to an increase in volume of distribution (amount of drug diluted in the total quantity of body water) of lipid soluble drugs and a reduction in the volume of distri-bution of water-soluble drugs such as digoxin and aminoglycosides. In order to achieve a therapeutic drug concentration, reduced doses of these drugs or low maintenance doses are required. Titrating doses of medicines also helps to prevent the development of adverse drug events (Leipzig, 1999; Cohen, 2000). In the older person, lipid soluble drugs may remain in fat deposit for prolonged periods of time. For example, benzodiazepines require an adequate time to reach the required concentration before increasing the dose. It should be remembered that lipid-soluble drugs may continue to exert their effect after the drug has been discontinued.

In the older person, the serum albumin concentration may be subject to reductions of 15–20%, particularly during periods of illness. Such reductions can impact on the binding of drugs that commonly bind to albumin such as warfarin and phenytoin. Consideration has to be given when measuring total drug levels which include both protein-bound and free drugs (Ericksson, 1984). When the albumin level is low, the fraction of free drug is increased. For example, warfarin is usually 99% bound to albumin, but when albumin levels are low the amount of free drug can be higher. This can lead to increased anticoagulant activity and toxicity (Schwartz, 1999).

Drug metabolism

Absorbed drugs will travel from the gut to the liver where they are metabolised to reduce their toxicity and to be excreted. Metabolism allows lipid-soluble drugs to be metabolised or converted to more water-soluble products in order to enhance their excretion, either via the urine or faeces, and removal from the body. The process of drug metabolism predominantly occurs in the liver, but it can also occur in the kidneys, adrenal glands, lungs, placenta, skin and the gut.

In the liver, drug metabolism involves two phases and two different groups of catalysing enzymes (see Figure 3.2). Usually drugs require both phases to complete their conversion to a water-soluble byproduct or metabolite that can then be excreted by the kidney. The metabolic reactions that occur during phase 1 involve a group of enzymes that are collectively referred to as cytochrome P450 (P stands for protein and 450 nm is the level of absorption determined by spectrophotometry). This enzyme system is located within the smooth endoplasmic reticulum and mitochrondrial cristae of the liver. Phase 1 metabolism can involve three distinct chemical reactions: oxidation, reduction and hydrolysis. The aim of these reactions is to chemically alter the structure of the drug to allow it to be recognised by the conjugation enzymes identified during Phase 2, and to make the drug water-soluble.

Absorbed drug → Phase 1 → oxidation + phase 2 → conjugation → drug elimination

Figure 3.2 The two phases of drug metabolism.

The second phase of metabolism involves a series of chemical reactions collectively referred to as conjugation reactions. These chemical reactions aim to make drugs/chemicals more water soluble and generally inactive, to facilitate their excretion via the kidney or the bile. Conjugation reactions occur within the cytoplasm of the hepatocyte and aim to increase the water solubility of the drug, rendering it available for excretion. The enzymes involved in these reactions include glycuronyl transferase and glutathione. Both are very important, as they help to detoxify drugs. For example, paracetamol is metabolised by cytochrome P450 during phase 1 and by glycuronyl transferase during phase 2. The metabolites or drug by-products are then excreted as mercapturic acid in the urine.

The first-pass effect or pre-systemic elimination is an important aspect of hepatic metabolism, as drugs that are taken orally can be excreted quickly with limited overall efficacy. The benefit of administering drugs by the per rectum route is that they avoid the first-pass effect. Many pharmaceutical companies acknowledge the importance of the first-pass effect when undertaking research with novel compounds and may manufacture new drugs that focus on this method of excretion.

Factors affecting drug metabolism

Variability is a serious problem when drugs are used clinically; it can result in lack of efficacy (therapeutic effectiveness) or lead to unexpected side effects. Individuals vary widely in their response to some drugs. Variability is categorised as variation in either drug disposition (pharmacokinetic variability) or in pharmacological response (pharmacodynamic variability). A range of factors are proposed which can influence both forms of variability: genetic (single gene effects, ethnic and sex differences), environmental effects (diet, concurrent drug ingestion or cigarette smoking) and pre-existing pathology (renal and hepatic disease or hormonal imbalance).

In terms of therapeutic effectiveness, drugs may vary due to extremes of age, as drugs can produce greater and prolonged effects in babies/neonates and the elderly. The age of the person can influence drug metabolism, drug excretion and renal function, drug sensitivity, and capacity to bind onto plasma proteins, in addition to having an effect on drug metabolism and drug excretion.

In the older person, phase one metabolism can decline as a result of reduced hepatic blood flow. Reductions of 50% of hepatic blood flow are often a consequence of reduced cardiac output (Beers, 1992). This may also cause atrophic changes within the liver, leading to reductions in size. The reduction in phase 1 metabolism can affect the metabolism of diazepam and flurazepam and prolong the duration of respective activity.

Table 3.1 Sites of metabolism and excretion of drugs.

Metabolism via the liver	Renal excretion
Erythromycin	Atenolol
Antidepressants	Ace inhibitors – captopril and enalapril
Calcium channel blockers	Digoxin
Hypnotics	Hydrocholorothiazide
Levodopa	Penicillins
Meteoprolol	Quinolones
Metronidazole	Lithium
Omprazole	Procainamide
Nitrates	
Warfarin	

It is important to remember that the metabolism and clearance of drugs via either the kidney or the liver can be affected by Cytochrome P450 enzyme inducers (drugs or agents that speed up the rate of drug metabolism) and enzyme inhibitors (drugs or agents that reduce the rate of drug metabolism) (Table 3.1). This fact should be taken into consideration when prescribing for older people, especially when the individual is prescribed multiple drugs.

The elimination half-life of a drug is the time it takes for the concentration of a drug to reduce by 50% following drug excretion. For each individual drug, the elimination half-life will differ. The elimination half-life of a drug is used as an estimate of the frequency by which drugs can be administered or the recommended dosing interval. Recommendations for the dosing intervals for drugs can be found in the British National Formulary, e.g. paracetamol can be prescribed 4–6 hourly. It is proposed that the effect of ageing increases the elimination half-life for several drugs (Schwartz, 1999).

Diet can also influence the metabolism and the resultant toxicity of the drug. For example, phenytoin is thought to reduce the absorption of intestinal calcium, thereby inducing osteoporosis, diets high in protein reduce the absorption of levodopa, consumption of green leafy vegetables diminishes the effectiveness of warfarin therapy (Dharmarajan & Ugalino, 2001) and grapefruit juice inhibits the metabolic actions of Cytochrome P450 3A4 and prolongs the affects of nifidipine and triazolam (Schwartz, 1999).

Drug excretion

Drugs can be excreted via the urinary or biliary system, resulting in the excretion of waste products either in the faeces or urine. Drugs predominantly select a main route of excretion (Table 3.1). The urinary system is by far the most common method of excretion, with up to 90% of drugs being excreted in the urine (Hämmerlein et al., 1998). Drugs are excreted via the urine using three main mechanisms: glomerular filtration, tubular reabsorption and tubular secretion.

Blood is filtered via the afferent tubule into the glomerulus, where it will reach Bowmans capsule. Bowmans capsule contains a series of capillaries that selectively filter drugs and alcohol according to their molecular weight. The capsule contains pores or podocytes that act as selective filters to prevent large molecules such as protein, sugars and plasma proteins from filtering through the membrane. This is a functional capacity that acts to filter drugs based on osmotic principle of particle transfer. Drugs that weigh greater than 20,000 Daltons or those bound to plasma proteins will be retained within the plasma and transported via the efferent arteriole to the proximal tubule. About 80% of drugs are reabsorbed in this way. Only 20% of drugs will be small enough to be selectively filtered by osmosis through the plasma membrane of Bowmans capsule. This property of particle transfer enables small molecules to maintain the renal threshold for protein, sugar and osmotic pressure. It is an essential prerequisite for renal homoestasis. This inability to pass through the membrane maintains the renal threshold for sugar at around 10mmol/L and prevents protein from also filtering through the membrane (Burke et al., 2003).

When drugs are excreted into the proximal tubule they are absorbed across the plasma membrane by way of carrier system transport. Unlike glomerular filtration, carrier mediated transport can achieve maximal drug clearance even when most of the drug is bound to plasma protein. For example, penicillin is about 80% bound to plasma proteins, therefore the drug is cleared very slowly by filtration but almost completely removed by proximal tubule secretion with a high overall rate of elimination. Carriers can transport drug molecules against an electrochemical gradient, therefore can reduce the plasma concentration to zero. Tubular secretion is potentially the most effective mechanism for drug elimination by the kidney, since 80% of the drug that is delivered to the kidney is presented to a carrier.

The renal tubules have a great ability to reabsorb water and electrolytes. Water-soluble drugs with low tubular permeability will be retained within the tubule, so the concentration may increase up to 100 times that of the urine. Most drugs are reabsorbed passively so the concentration of drug is relevant to the plasma and to the solute. The nephron is actively involved in sodium (Na^+) transport. Mechanisms that control Na^+Cl^- (sodium chloride) and water balance generally involve circa 99% of the Na^+ being filtered and reabsorbed. Remaining cations (positively charged molecules) are removed as water is reabsorbed. Remaining solutes are progressively dragged along the nephron.

In the distal tubule, drugs that are highly lipid-soluble will be excreted slowly or reabsorbed across the plasma membrane and redistributed within the circulation. These drugs would then be refiltered/ metabolised in an attempt to excrete them.

Biliary excretion

Drugs are transferred from the plasma to the liver via the biliary system. Bile is formed in the liver hepatocytes and is then secreted in a Na/K ATPase controlled environment between the basolateral membrane and the liver sinusoidal lining cells. Bile is drained from the liver via bile ducts to the common bile duct where it is modified by the gut hormones and is the main route of excretion of cholesterol, bilirubin, sex and adrenal hormones and thyroxine. Drugs are transferred from the plasma to the liver where biliary acids play a key role in conjugation reaction. Conjugated drugs are transferred to the intestine, where hydrolysis takes place before the drug is excreted via the faeces, e.g. rifampicin is absorbed in the gut, undergoes a conjugation reaction in the liver and is then excreted in the faeces. Similarly, morphine, chloramphenicol, stilboestrol and digoxin are excreted in the faeces following conjugation reactions.

Drugs can also be recycled between the gut and the liver by a process involving the enterohepatic circulation, often referred to as enterohepatic recycling. This process accounts for about 20% of circulating drugs that are excreted via the biliary system. The active drug is released then reabsorbed as it is transported through the enterohepatic recirulation or liver and intestine circulation. Gut bacteria contain drug-metabolising enzymes called α-glycones which reverse the metabolic changes that the drug had undergone and convert the drug back to its original chemical structure. The drug is then reabsorbed in the liver where the process of metabolism will recommence. For example, digoxin binds to cholesytramine and is then reabsorbed within the terminal ileum and excreted in the bile to undergo recycling. Digoxin normally has a plasma half-life of 11.5 days, but as a result of enterohepatic recycling this figure is increased to 66 days.

Drug excretion is reduced by 50–70% in older people (Aronson, 1999). The kidney is subjected to age-related changes involving decreased blood flow and a 30% reduction in renal mass. The glomerular filtration rate (GFR) is calculated using the measurement of creatinine clearance (Taffet, 1999) that is then used as an assessment of renal function (Gleason, 1996). Cockcroft and Gault (1976) suggest that creatinine clearance should be calculated prior to prescribing drugs for the older person. Reports vary with regard to the impact of ageing on creatinine clearance. Jackson (1995) states that there is no change in creatinine clearance, whereas Taffet (1999) proposes that there is a reduction of 10 ml/min per decade due to reduced blood flow to the kidneys and a reduction in renal mass.

Table 3.2 Impact of age on pharmacokinetic parameters.

Pharmacokinetic process	Resultant effect
Drug distribution	Decrease in total body water Increase in fat compartment (adipose tissue) Decrease in muscle mass
Protein binding	Reduction in serum albumin often associated with liver disease
Drug metabolism	Reduced number of hepatocytes due to reduced size of the liver Decrease in hepatic blood flow Reductions in phase 1 metabolism
Drug excretion	Reductions in the size of the kidney mainly involving the renal cortex Reduced renal blood flow Reductions in creatinine clearance by 1 ml/min occur from 30 years of age onwards. Decline in tubular secretion

Alterations in pharmacokinetic parameters caused by changes in hepatic homeostasis and the decline in drug clearance and polypharmacy render older people susceptible to adverse drug events (Hämmerlein et al., 1998; Cooper, 1999; Ford, 2000; Leipzig, 2000) and unplanned hospitalisation (Bero, et al., 1991). Older people are three times more likely to develop an adverse reaction to a drug than individuals who are in the third decade of life. Adverse drug events can be prevented by titrating the dose of drug, prescribing at the lowest dose possible (Cohen, 2000), maintaining appropriate prescribing practice and undertaking medication review (Rochon & Gurwitz, 1999; Naugler, 2000; Walley & Scott, 1995; Sheenhan & Feely, 1999).

In summary, the body responds to the actions of drugs via the processes of drug absorption, drug distribution, drug metabolism and drug excretion. Table 3.2 provides an outline of how each process can be influenced by the events of ageing (see Figure 3.3).

Pharmacodynamics

Pharmacodynamics is the influence of the drug on the body. The drug will produce a physiological response before being excreted via the kidneys or faeces (see Figure 3.3).

Drugs are manufactured with an intended mode of action. Most drugs are effective because they bind to particular target proteins: enzymes, carriers, ion channels and receptors.

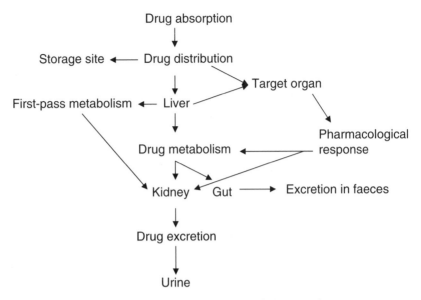

Figure 3.3 Interplay between pharmacokinetic and pharmacodynamic processes.

Enzymes

Enzymes are catalysts that aid the speed of a reaction without themselves being consumed. Enzymes recognise and respond to molecules called substrates that can bind specifically to their active sites either by a lock and key mechanism, where the substrate fits comfortably within the active site, or by 'induced fit' mechanism, which allows the enzyme and substrate to form complexes. As a result, the substrate is catabolised during the reaction. Drugs which act on enzymes usually act by inhibition and involve short-term reactions. Typical examples of drugs that act as enzymic inhibitors include: COX II inhibitors, ACE inhibitors, aspirin, NSAIDs and theophylline.

Carrier molecules

Transport of small molecules such as glucose, choline, amino acids and physiological ions such as sodium (Na^+) and calcium (Ca^{2+}) generally requires a carrier protein due to the fact that ions and small molecules are generally insufficiently lipid-soluble to penetrate the lipid membrane. Carrier proteins have a recognition site that makes them specific for a particular molecule and also drug targets. Examples of drugs that use carrier proteins to access cells include tricyclic antidepressants and cocaine.

Ion channels

Ion channels are the simplest form of drug target. Ion channels are proteins that are embedded within the plasma membrane of cells and act by permitting the transport of ions across the membrane. The most common ions that are involved are sodium (Na^+), calcium (Ca^{2+}) and potassium (K^+). Drugs that interact with ion channels physically block the channel and prevent the movement of ions across the plasma membrane. Common examples of ion channel blockers include the diuretic amiloride, which acts by the blocking of Na^+ entry into the renal tubular cell. Calcium channels can be categorised according to the location and type of ion channel: L-type Ca^{2+} channels such as are found on muscle cells or the T-type found on nerve cell. Nifedipine is a common example of L-type Ca^{2+} channel blocker. Potassium channels are also used as targets for drug action such as glipizide and glibenclamide, which act to regulate ATP-dependent K^+ channels within the pancreas. These ion channels help to maintain the regulation of insulin release from the pancreas in diabetic patients.

Receptor operated channels

Receptor operated channels are involved in controlling the action of various smooth muscle contracting agents, for example noradrenalin, and acetylcholine and also gamma aminobutyric acid (GABA). These channels respond to changes in specific ions such as Ca^{2+}, chloride (Cl^-) or K^+. GABA is an amino acid formed from glutamate which acts as a central nervous system (CNS) transmitter. GABA receptors regulate the conductance of numerous ions which control the homeostasis of neurons within the CNS. Benzodiazepine tranquillisers act to facilitate the opening of the GABA channel and by doing so cause a change in shape of the receptor and exert a sedatory effect on the patient.

Ligand-gated ion channels

Ligands are small molecules which are structurally similar to the normal chemical/hormone/agonist that occupies the receptor. These open when their associated receptor is occupied by an agonist (neurotransmitter, e.g. adrenaline). Cimetidine is a common example of a ligand; it is structurally similar to histamine which blocks the transport of histamine across the H_2 receptor in the parietal cell of the fundus of the stomach and so reduces the secretion of hydrochloric acid.

Receptors

Receptors are proteins that are embedded within the plasma membrane of cells. Their function is to assist chemical communication within the cell and act as part of the signal transduction mechanisms that regulate cell activity. There are more than 32 different types of receptor, which may be subdivided as follows.

Fast transmitter receptors

Fast transmitter receptors are directly linked to ion channels such as Cl^-, e.g. GABA receptors and also G protein-coupled receptors. These are a family of receptors that belong to 5HT, adrenergic and dopamine receptors. G proteins are 'go-between' proteins which interact with guanine nucleotides, guanosine diphosphate (GDP) and guanosine triphosphate (GTP) and play a key role in the communication or signal transduction (chemical communication) mechanisms between the receptor, cellular enzymes such as protein kinases and the nucleus of the cell.

Hormone and slow transmitter receptors (muscarinic acetlycholine receptor)

Receptors respond to chemical messengers or hormones such as histamine and neurotransmitters such as acetylcholine and adrenaline. A neurotransmitter acts on the post-synaptic membrane of a nerve or muscle cell and transiently increases its permeability to a particular ion, e.g. acetylcholine at the neurotransmitter junction can increase the permeability of Na^+/K^+ ions. The inward current of Na^+ generates the action potential. The concentration of the transmitter reaches a peak in a microsecond, then decays as the influx of ions reaches 10^7/microsec. The cell then returns to a resting state until the next influx of ions triggers the release of the neurotransmitter.

Insulin and growth factors receptors

Insulin and growth factors receptors are directly linked to tyrosine kinase to mediate the reactions of a variety of growth factors, peptide mediators and insulin.

Steroid receptors

Steroid receptors are soluble cytosolic membrane or intranuclear proteins which strongly bind to nuclear chromatin (genetic material). Steroid molecules cross the lipid membrane and bind to the receptor, which unfolds and exposes the DNA and starts to control the regulation of DNA replication within the cell nucleus. The actions of steroids are generally very slow, so responses can take weeks to months to show a determined effect. Common examples are inhaled steroids such as beclamethosone and fluticasone used in the treatment of asthma.

Receptor agonism

An agonist is a drug that mimics the effects of a neurotransmitter or hormone or alters the physiology of a cell by binding to the plasma membrane or intracellular receptors. Salbutamol is a B_2 agonist that mimics the actions of isoprenaline and adrenaline which normally circulate within the lungs following release by sympathetic nerve terminals. Isoprenaline and adrenaline cause bronchodilation of smooth muscle cells within the bronchus. Salbutamol mimics these actions by relaxing bronchiolar smooth muscle cells. The potency of an agonist depends on the affinity (ability to enhance once bound) and efficacy (changes which lead to the effect required).

Antagonists act in the opposite manner to agonists; their intention is to inhibit or block the binding of the agonist to the receptor site. Antagonists compete with agonists for the receptor site in cells. Antagonists will have a structural affinity with the receptor to allow it to compete with the agonist for the binding site on the receptor, but will not produce any other physical change. For example, atrovent is a muscarinic antagonist which competitively inhibits the binding of acetylcholine at the receptor site. In doing so, atrovent will prevent acetylcholine-induced bronchospasm in asthmatic patients.

Pharmacodynamics and the effects of ageing

With age, older people become increasingly vulnerable to the effects of drugs and are likely to develop organ disease which merits treatment with a variety of medicines (Beers, 1997) (Table 3.3). Organ disease may increase the likelihood of a patient developing an adverse reaction to a drug. For example, patients being treated for depression with concomitant glaucoma may find that the anticholinergic effects of the

Table 3.3 Factors that increase the risk of drug-related mortality and morbidity in the older person.

Factor	Consequence
Pharmacokinetic effects	Reductions in lean muscle mass Increased adipose tissue Reduced renal and hepatic function
Pharmacodynamic effects	Impaired homeostatic mechanisms Increased sensitivity to the actions of drugs
Existing pathologies	Disease medicine interactions Multiple pathologies requiring pharmacological treatment
Cognitive impairment	Memory loss, incipient dementia, poor adherence to medication regimens
Physical status	Problems with manual dexterity, vision and hearing that impact on adherence to medication

antidepressants cause an increase in intraocular pressure (Roberts & Tumer, 1988). The anticholinergic effects of tricyclic antidepressants can also lead to urinary retention, blurred vision and confusion in older people (Sheehan & Feely, 1999). The use of these categories of drugs should be routinely reviewed (DoH, 2001, 2001a).

Dharmarajan and Ugalino (2001) suggest that the effects of ageing may lead to reductions or increments in receptor sensitivity which impact on the ability of the body to respond to drugs, e.g. ß-adrenergic activity diminishes with age, therefore patients administering either ß agonists or ß antagonists may require larger doses to produce a response. In contrast, older people are more sensitive to the actions of opiates and benzodiazepines, which results in an increase in the development of side effects. This may be related to blunted homoestatic mechanisms whereby the individual develops sedation, respiratory depression or constipation, especially if drug doses are not titrated to meet the needs of the older patient (Table 3.4). Numerous drugs have been shown to possess a variety of actions which can pose problems for the older person. Common examples are aspirin and benzodiazepine. Aspirin exerts its antipyretic, anti-inflammatory, anti-thrombotic

Table 3.4 Medicines that can be potentially harmful to the older person.

Medicine	Effect
Antibiotics, e.g. sulphamethoxazole/ trimethoprim	Idiosyncratic variation increases the risk of type B adverse drug reactions. Treatment for urinary tract infections can be problematic
Anticoagulants	Treatment with warfarin increases the risk of drug interactions. There is also the risk of haemorrhage
Antihypertensive agents	Large doses of diuretics can induce hypotensive events, dehydration and electrolyte imbalance. There is a need to observe for ceiling dose effects with thiazides, and monitor electrolytes
Digoxin	Narrow therapeutic index and decreased clearance increase risk of blurred vision, nausea, vomiting, arrhythmias. Drug and potassium monitoring required
Non-steroidal anti-inflammatory agents	Risk of gastric ulceration, renal impairment and exacerbation of hypertension
Psychoactive agents (antidepressants, sedatives, antipsychotics, hypnotics)	Can induce anticholinergic effects, e.g. agitation, confusion, impaired vision, urinary retention, constipation, postural hypotension, problems concentrating

and analgesic properties through enzyme inhibition of mediators (biochemicals) produced during the inflammatory response. Similarly, benzodiazepine tranquillisers bind to the benzodiazepine receptor sub-units of the γ-aminobutyric (GABA) receptor potentiating its inhibitory actions and can therefore exert sedative, anti-anxiety and antiepleptic actions. In the older person, there is an increased sensitivity to opiates, benzodiazepines, ß-blockers, central a-agonists and tricyclic anti-depressants due to atherosclerosis induced narrowing of carotid and vertebral arteries (Larsson et al., 1987).

Older patents prescribed calcium channel blockers such as nife-dipine, verapamil and dilitiazem for the treatment of hypertension may be predisposed to postural hypotension, falls and confusion due to impaired baroreceptor reflexes (Roberts & Tumer, 1988; Sheehan & Feely, 1999). When calcium channel blockers are used in combination with digoxin, they have been shown to raise the serum levels of digoxin (Eriksson, 1984). This can be dangerous as older people are more prone to the toxic effects of digoxin due to altered tissue sensitivity or decreased glomerular filtration rate (GFR). Digoxin toxicity can manifest itself in raised serum drug levels, electrolyte disturbances involving hypokalaemia, hypomagnesaemia and hy-percalcemia, which impact on the sensitivity of the myocardium to the drug.

Drugs interactions with verapamil and diuretics can also induce toxicity which could manifest itself by nausea and vomiting, photopho-bia, confusion, arrhythmias such as bradycardia and ventricular and atrial ectopic beats, ventricular tachycardias and abnormal atrioven-tricular conduction. These drugs should be prescribed at the lowest possible dose (Dartnell et al., 1996).

Elderly patients prescribed diuretics are prone to the side effects, which include urinary incontinence, hyperuricaemia, postural hypo-tension and hypokalaemia (Moore et al., 1998). In cases where a com-bination of a thiazide and a potassium sparing diuretic is used, this combination can increase the risk of hyperkalaemia in the older person (Cunningham et al., 1997).

It is known that anticoagulation with warfarin can reduce the incidence of stroke in patients with atrial fibrillation (Honer & Lancaster, 1996). Careful consideration should be given when prescrib-ing warfarin for older people as they are more sensitive to the actions of the drug and therefore can be maintained on lower doses of the drug (Walley & Scott, 1995). Prescribers should be aware of the possibility of drug interactions when prescribing warfarin with co-trimoxazole, omperazaole, cimetidine or NSAIDs as these can initiate bleeding (Honer & Lancaster, 1996) or bleeding complications (Gleason, 1996).

Adverse drug interactions may arise as a consequence of inappro-priate prescribing due to the incorporation of inadequate dosing protocols and inappropriate medication management review, or as a consequence of patients' demands (Walley & Scott, 1995; Moore et al., 2001). In order to reduce the risks associated with the development of drug interactions, prescribers should consider the use of prescribing indicators to assist prescribing practice (Knight & Avorn 2001; Osborne & Batty, 1997). Prescribing indicators can be used as a checklist to assist nurse prescribers and community matrons when prescribing medication to older people. Assess the patient for the following:

- the accuracy of documentation of patient education and the prescribed medication
- the currency of the medications prescribed and the efficacy of prescribed medication
- therapeutic drug monitoring of patients receiving warfarin and diuretics therapies, and renal function tests for patients on ACE inhibitors
- the avoidance of the use of chloropropamide in older people due to risk of hypoglycaemia
- the avoidance of the use of cholinergic antagonists due to risk of confusion and barbiturate therapy due to risk of falls
- polypharmacy and quantity of generic and as-required drugs prescribed
- the number of patients prescribed duplicated drugs (H_2 receptor antagonists and proton-pump inhibitors)
- the frequency of prescription of digoxin with/without anticoagulant/or aspirin
- the frequency of ß$_2$ agonists prescribed with or without steroids and ACE
- inhibitors with potassium sparing diuretics
- appropriateness of prescribed benzodiazepines.

Conclusion

Pharmacology is a complex subject which is underpinned by knowledge of applied physiology of the liver, kidney and gastrointestinal tract and organ-specific pathophysiology. In order to prescribe competently, the prescriber should possess a working knowledge of these scientific areas, in addition to a good understanding of the impact of ageing in the older person and its influence on both pharmacokinetic and pharmacodynamic parameters, including a working knowledge of adverse drug events and how to prevent them. Prescribing for older people is a complex task that requires adroitness and a comprehensive knowledge of medicines and their actions (Thompson & Crome, 2002). The use of prescribing indicators can assist this process.

Implications for practice

- Nurses, nurse prescribers and community matrons require a working knowledge of applied pharmacology and therapeutics with specific reference to the impact of ageing on pharmacological parameters.
- Nurse prescribers and community matrons should be aware of the potential problems of prescribing for older people and the need to give careful consideration to high-risk medications and employ prescribing indicators in order to regulate their prescribing practice.
- Nurse prescribers and community matrons managing the care of older people with long-term conditions need to constantly update their knowledge of medicines that they regularly prescribe and monitor older people for adverse drug reactions.

Medication management and the older person

Maggi Banning

Learning objectives

The aim of this chapter is to introduce the reader to the concept of medication management. This chapter will contain the following:

- an overview of the patient-centred medication review
- an introduction to the single assessment process
- an overview of medication review
- a summary of the role of health care professionals in medication review
- principles of prescribing for older people
- a summary of rational prescribing and prescribing support.

Introduction

Medication management is a complex process which has been the subject of reviews (DoH, 2002a), several white papers (DoH, 2001, 2001a, 2004), and a collaboration project between medical and pharmacy colleagues (RCGP, 2000; Bernett et al., 2003). The Pharmaceutical Association defines medication management (NPA, 1998, p. 7) as a process which:

'covers the processes and support system which are available to help people who self-administer their medication in the community to gain the optimum health benefit from their prescription. It happens after medication has been dispensed, in the person's own home or in a homely

setting. It may involve input from home care workers, family carers and health or social care professionals whom the person encounters in the course of their care.'

According to the Royal Pharmaceutical Society of Great Britain (RPSGB, 2003) medication management is a broad term that encompasses several interrelated issues including:

- patient-centred medication review, to assess adverse effects and compliance
- rational prescribing and prescribing support
- repeat prescribing
- patient information
- access to medicines
- improvements at the primary and secondary care interface.

The importance of medication management has gradually increased because of its multi-focal nature and role in the care of older people. The growing interest in medication management was influenced by the quantity of older people receiving medicines to manage their pathological conditions, many of which are long-term conditions, the ever-increasing rise in unplanned admission to hospital in people of older age and the escalating financial costs to the health service. It is suggested that 50% of NHS expenditure is spent prescribing for older people and about 6–10% of this cost is related to drug wastage (Oboh, 2006). Roughly 36% of older people routinely administer four or more medicines (Oboh, 2006) and about 50% of older people fail to administer their drugs as prescribed (Medicines Partnership, 2002). It is not just the quantity of medicines being administered on a daily basis that is important, but also the difficulties that can arise from the administration of medicines. The need for medication management is also supported by the high incidence of unplanned hospital admissions (6–17%) in the older people category (DoH, 2001a). Of these, 10% of unplanned admissions may relate to the inability of older people to effectively manage their medicines (Oboh, 2006).

The NSF for Older People: Medicines and Older People (DoH, 2001a) identified several medication issues as problem areas, including:

- polypharmacy
- non-compliance with drug regimens due to patients' failure to understand their medicines and not taking them as prescribed (RCP, 1997)
- inappropriate prescribing of long-term drugs
- incidence of side effects such as falls, gastro-intestinal bleeding or the development of congestive heart failure (Feder et al., 2000)
- inadequate monitoring of clinical and biochemical indicators.

These issues were among the determining factors that instigated the development of the medication management pilot schemes implemented by the National Prescribing Centre in 2003. This scheme was operationalised in four stages throughout the UK and involved the participation of a selection of community pharmacists (NPC, 2003). The scheme has subsequently been successfully rolled out throughout the UK.

Although medication management is part of pharmaceutical care, it is also an issue for primary care professionals and involves everyone who takes medicines and families, carers and friends who care for people requiring treatment for long-term conditions. The concept of medication management is briefly introduced in nurse prescribing education and training programmes but is lacking in pre-registration nurse programmes. This issue needs to be addressed, especially if qualified nurses take on medication management roles. In addition, role preparation courses, such as for the role of community matron, need to include instruction on all key aspects of medication management (see Figure 4.1).

Medication review and the older person

In 2001, the NSF for Older People set out a programme of action and reform to address the failure to meet the medication management needs of older people. This concept was supported by the need for older people to gain maximum benefit from their medicines so that they do not suffer from medication-related unwanted side effects. This should be the 'overall goal of any medicines management service that is delivered to older people' (Oboh, 2006, p. 206).

In delivering the NSF for Older People (DoH, 2001), specific targets were set for primary care. These included a target that by 2002, all older people aged 75 years and over taking medicines should have an annual medication review. For patients who administer four or more medicines, this review should be held on a six-monthly basis. By 2004, primary care organisations should have schemes in place that enabled older people to obtain help regarding their medicines from a qualified community pharmacist (DoH, 2001).

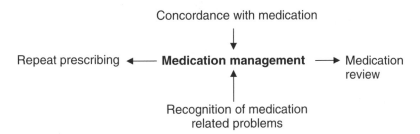

Figure 4.1 Outline of factors central to medication management.

Medication review may be defined as 'a structured, critical examination of a patient's medicines with the objective of reaching an agreement with the patient about treatment, optimising the use of medicines, and minimising the number of medication related problems and reducing waste' (Medicines Partnership, 2002).

That the need for medication review is emerging as an essential component of medicines management has been illustrated in numerous policy documents, such as the NSF for Older People (DoH, 2001) and the introduction of the single assessment process (DoH, 2001a), and the annual health check for older people (GMSC, 1989) is a GP requirement for qualifying for sustained quality allowance (DoH, 2002).

According to the Medicines Partnership (2002), the frequency of the review process is dependent on the patient, their condition and the complexity of their needs. Independent of the patient and resources available, the following underlying principles of medication review should be adhered to:

- all patients should have a chance to raise questions and highlight their needs about their medicines
- medication review seeks to improve or optimise impact of treatment for the individual patient
- the review is undertaken in a systematic way, by a competent person
- any changes resulting from the review are agreed with the patient
- the review is documented in the patient's notes
- the impact of any change is monitored.

The process of the review may include an assessment of the patient's lists of medicines and scrutinising these to identify anomalies and problems by referring to the patient's records and by assessing the appropriateness of the drug regimen in relation to the patient's condition and history (Medicines Partnership, 2002). The focus of a medication review is on the drugs that the patient actually takes rather than what are prescribed, and what effect the drugs are having on the condition being treated, e.g. worsening or improving the condition and also if there are any additional medical needs. The patient consultation provides opportunities to discuss indirectly the patient's beliefs and any lifestyle changes that have been necessary with regard to routinely taking medicines (Medicines Partnership, 2002).

Medication review structure

The central focus of patient-centred medication review is the identification of health and social problems following the initial patient assessment (Oboh, 2006). The importance of older people complying with the medication review is discussed in the NSF for Older People (DoH, 2001). A key feature of the review process is patient participation in all decision-making related to the role of medicines in the management of their condition (Medicines Partnership, 2002).

Medication reviews are routinely carried out by General Practitioners (GPs), community matrons and in some cases nurse practitioners, community matrons and community pharmacists. Pharmacy driven medication review has been undertaken in day centres, care homes, community pharmacy, patients' homes and intermediate care centres (Oboh, 2006).

Community pharmacists were chosen to offer 'brown bag' schemes whereby people over the age of 65 years who were receiving treatment for long-term conditions and concurrently administering more than four medicines, were invited to visit their local pharmacy for a review of their medicines. Pharmacists consulted with older people on the usefulness of medicines prescribed in the management of major conditions. Pharmacists were able to detect the development of adverse effects that were associated with the medicines that were prescribed, and also reviewed medicines that were not efficacious. In some cases, older people were administering duplicate medicines, e.g. administering two NSAIDs that were not required.

The involvement of the pharmacist can produce marked improvements in the quality of medication management for older people (Neary, 2002; Schweizer & Hughes, 2001; Zermansky et al., 2001), particularly in relation to the treatment of depression and dementia (Mental Health Foundation, 2001, 2004).

Although GPs, community matrons, pharmacists and nurse practitioners may select to consult with patients 75 years and over or those concurrently administering more than four medicines, other select groups of older people who fall into specific categories include the following:

- residents of care homes
- individuals with sensory impairment such as poor sight or hearing difficulties
- people recently discharged from hospital with complex medicines
- people taking medicines that require special monitoring (e.g. lithium), or medicines with a wide range of side effects (e.g. NSAIDs) or a narrow therapeutic range (e.g. digoxin)
- people receiving medicines from more than one source (e.g. hospital specialist) and a general practitioner
- people who have had significant alterations to their drug regimen in the past three months
- people who may be suspected of being non-complaint with their medication

- individuals with mental states such as confusion, anxiety, depression or serious mental health problems
- individuals with symptoms that are indicative of an adverse drug reaction.

Health care professionals can track progress in medication review by considering the following:

- number of completed reviews at each level
- percentage of patients over the age of 75 years whose notes contain documented evidence of a medication review over the past 12 months
- percentage of patients 75 years and over concurrently administering four or more drugs who had received a medication review in the past 6 months
- percentage of vulnerable patients discharged from hospital on repeat medicines whose notes contain evidence of medication review within an 8-week period
- patient satisfaction with the medication review process
- estimated cost savings or cost increase from medication review.

The central focus of patient-centred medication review involves the identification of medication issues and the assessment of possible adverse effects and concerns regarding the concordance with medication. This can be achieved through the single assessment process.

The single assessment process

The single assessment process (SAP) 'is a collection of activities designed to assess and deal with older people's health and social care needs' (Medicines Partnership, 2002). The SAP is a patient-centred activity that allows opportunities for the individual to express their concerns about their medicines with the aim of improving concordance with prescribed medication (Medicines Partnership, 2002).

The importance of the single assessment process (SAP) and medication review in the older person has been highlighted in the NHS Plan (DoH, 2000), the NSF for Older People (DoH, 2001) and the NSF Medicines and Older People (DoH, 2001a). Standard 2 of the National Service Framework for Older People emphasises the importance of 'person-centred care' and states that:

> *'NHS and social care services treat older people as individuals and enable them to make choices about their own care. This is achieved through the single assessment process integrated commissioning arrangements and integrated provision of services, including community equipment and continence services.'* (DoH, 2001).

The purpose of SAP is to 'ensure that older people receive appropriate, effective and timely responses to their health and social care needs, and that professional resources are used effectively' (LOPSDP, 2003, p. 1). SAP is regarded as the central method of identifying the health and social care needs of older people by pharmacists (Mental Health Foundation, 2004; Oboh, 2006).

The SAP contains several important interrelated components which are essential to the process (Medicines Partnership, 2002). These include the following:

- the individual lies at the heart of the assessment and care planning
- SAPs are timed in accordance with the needs of the individual
- the provision of service delivered is subjected to formalised care planning procedures that are recorded and updated as necessary
- all patient information is collated, shared and stored as effectively as possible.

Professionals involved in the SAP are expected to work effectively, contribute to the assessment process and manage the care provided with the assistance of care managers.

There are four levels of assessment in the SAP. Each level has a different responsibility and aim, to ensure that people receive the care needed appropriate to their individual needs. These are contact assessment, overview assessment, specialist assessment and comprehensive assessment.

During the contact assessment, the older person is assessed when their needs appear to be significant. The contact assessment will involve the attainment of basic information on the potential problem, wider social and health care needs and family and carer support systems available to the patient, and will include the identification of possible solutions. This form of assessment usually takes place in the GP surgery when the patient registers for assessment and treatment. This form of patient assessment will be undertaken by a competent professional who should have received adequate education and training in the assessment of older people.

Overview assessment is used when the health care professional feels that a more detailed assessment is required. This form of assessment will include four trigger questions (see next section). The assessor should be trained to use the four questions and know how to respond to the patients' responses. A nurse or pharmacist may undertake this form of review.

The specialist assessment is used to explore patients' specific needs in relation to medication management. This process should examine causation and presence of a health-related problem that is linked to the patient's existing illness. This form of assessment is undertaken by a specialist assessor or competent health care professional and involves the use of an in-depth medication assessment tool to assess the patient's needs.

The final form of SAP assessment is the comprehensive assessment. This involves all domains of the SAP. Older people in this category may require an intensive and prolonged level of support that can be achieved by either intermediate care or permanent admission to a care home. In this instance, the health care professional may also recruit the help of a psychologist who specialises in geriatric medicine. In this form of SAP, the assessments undertaken should be co-ordinated, with final analyses drawn together to form a reasonable solution.

Trigger questions

A key component of the SAP is the use of trigger questions to assist non-medically qualified individuals to perform assessments, such as people from the voluntary organisations (Medicines Partnership, 2002). Four trigger questions were developed by the London Pharmacy Service. The questions focused on issues of access, compliance and concordance, day-to-day medicines management and clinical issues. The key questions were as follows:

- Do you need help getting a regular supply of your medicines? Yes/no
- Do you always take your medicines the way your doctor wants you to? Yes/no
- Can you get all of your medicines out of their containers? Yes/no
- Do you think realistically that some of your medicines could work better? Yes/no

A function on the SAP is to use the four trigger questions to identify patients who have health and social care needs. In response to the questions, patients may be asked a series of link questions, for example:

Do you need help getting a regular supply of your medicines?
Patients who respond yes will then be asked the following questions:
What type of help is needed? Does this help include any of the following:
Help getting to and from the surgery/pharmacy
A prescription collection and delivery service from the pharmacy
Help arranging to get all your medicines at the same time
Help remembering to take your medicines regularly
Other?

Do you always take your medicines the way your doctor wants you to?
A 'no' response will trigger the question, what causes the person to
take them differently? In response to this the assessor may ask any
of the following link questions. Is this related to:
Being unsure how the doctor wants me to take them
Don't understand the directions
Don't take some medicines at all (stopped taking them)
Get side effects from medicines
Adjust the dose sometimes myself
Share medicines with other people
Lost faith in the medicines?

Can you get all of your medicines out of their containers?
If no, why not. Do you suffer from any of the following:
Arthritis, stroke, tremor, lack of strength, lack of dexterity
Difficulty with blister packs, poor eyesight, can't manage child resis-
tant closures
Can't manage a particular dose form (e.g. inhaler)?

**Do you/ think realistically that some of your medicines could work
better?**
If yes, why?
Get side effects
Don't need to take some of the medicines now (symptoms have
resolved).
Medicines don't give immediate benefit
My illness has got worse
I still get symptoms even when I take my medicines
I need to purchase additional medicines from my community
pharmacy/chemist.

Care plans

As part of the SAP, the assessor will develop a comprehensive and
explicit care plan in agreement with the patient. This patient-centred
process aims to assess and develop a plan of care that meets the needs
of the individual. During the process of compiling a care plan the assessor should consider the age of the individual, geographic issues, culture,
faith, personal relationships, lifestyle choices and gender. All of these
issues can impact on the development of a programme of care that suits
the individual.

In preparing a care plan, the assessor should include the
following:

- a summary of identified needs that illustrate their intensity, any accompanying risks and potential for rehabilitation
- current objectives and anticipated outcomes for users
- a brief account of how services will impact on identified needs
- user involvement and contribution to the development of the plan
- a summary of what support the users require
- an account of the level and frequency of help that is to be provided
- a description of the monitoring processes involved
- name of care assessor.

Reviews should be scheduled to take place on a three-monthly basis. The review should evaluate whether the level and frequency of support is adequate to meet the needs of the individual and also reassess whether there has been a change in the ongoing needs. During this time, the assessor can also discuss any changes in the individual's personal, social and health needs and whether additional services are required. The care plan can then be amended as needed.

Health care professional involvement

A key aspect of SAP is that non-medically qualified individuals may participate in the assessment process. It has been shown that nurses and pharmacists can be influential, and comply with the SAP following the appropriate education and training. The success of the process is underpinned by the ability of assessors to comprehend the principles behind the four trigger questions, as each question has an underpinning meaning. In addition, the assessor should comprehend the significance of legal and ethical issues pertinent to the supply and administration of drugs.

Findings from the LOPSDP study indicate that during the SAP, nurse and pharmacist professionals differ in the form of medication-related problems they raise. For example, pharmacists tend to raise questions regarding access to medication and compliance of patients to their medication regimens. In contrast, district nurses will raise questions that are of a clinical nature. This apparent difference in the types of questions raised appears to be discipline-specific, which may be a consequence of the nature of previous professional training. This is an issue that needs to be addressed in the current education and training programme. Care assessor co-ordinators who manage the assessors undertaking the SAP process should also be aware of the possible tendency for discipline-specific awareness among assessors and the need for assessors to be fully complacent with all elements of the SAP process.

Nurses, community matrons and pharmacists may benefit from the guidance that can be offered from more experienced assessors. Gilbert

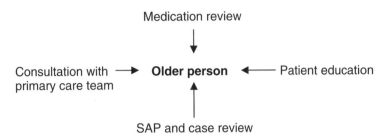

Figure 4.2 Role of health care professionals in the medication management of patients with long-term conditions.

et al. (2002) reported that 81% of mediation-related problems were ameliorated following interaction between the pharmacist and the GP. Although the GP's role is crucial, it has been suggested that many GPs prefer a less in-depth approach to medication management (Carter, 2004). This may be due to experience and use of prototypes that influence the clinical reasoning strategies employed during clinical assessment. Even so, it is essential that GPs provide instruction and guidance to inexperienced prescribers and community matrons, especially related to the prescribing of medicines for older people.

Prescribing practice

Recent developments in prescribing practice indicate that all independent prescribers will soon be authorised to prescribe all the medicines in the BNF with the exception of opioids (DOH, 2005c). This change in regulation will allow nurse and pharmacy prescribers and community matrons with an appropriate prescribing quaification to independently prescribe medicines to treat long-term conditions and manage the care of older people. This may mean that nurse prescribers may be involved in the SAP and medication review. This will require closer working relationships with community pharmacists and GPs and the need for prescribers to familiarise themselves with the principles of prescribing for the older person and to develop expertise in the medication management and medication education of older people (see Figure 4.2).

Principles of prescribing for the older person

There are several principles that the prescriber and community matron need to take into consideration when prescribing for the older person, including:

- Know the diagnosis and make sure that the prescriber, either nurse or pharmacist, has fully investigated the patient's case history and taken an accurate past medical history from the patient. This medical history should be supported with a full physical examination, and appropriate biochemical testing before prescribing any medication.

- Conduct a regular review of medication with the patient. It is necessary to explore the extent to which the patient is concordant with their current medication. Request that the patient brings their current medication to the consultation. In this way the nurse or nurse prescriber can ask the patient which medicines they regularly administer and whether the patient has developed any side effects from the medication. This will allow the nurse/nurse prescriber or community matron to ask whether the patient has any concerns regarding the medicines they are prescribed.

- Apply the principles of careful prescribing and do not prescribe medication when in doubt. Always seek a second opinion when there is any uncertainty. When prescribing medicines for older people always use the minimal dose required; as people increase in age it is necessary to reduce or titrate the dose of medicines that are excreted by the renal system, e.g. atenolol, captopril, digoxin, pencillins, hydrochlorothiazide, lithium and quinolones. This is because renal function starts to decline from the third decade of life (Dharmarajan & Ugalino, 2001). So by the time the person is in their sixth or seventh decade of life, residual renal function will have reduced quite dramatically.

- Be confident in their knowledge of medicines that they prescribe regularly. It is of utmost importance that the nurse prescriber has a working knowledge of pharmacodynamics and pharmacokinetic parameters before prescribing any medicine to the older person. This is essential as older people are more prone to the adverse effects of medicines, for example, medicines that may interact, such as phenytoin, digoxin, warfarin, amiodarone, selective serotonin re-uptake inhibitors such as fluoxetine and paroxetine and medicines with anticholinergic effects such as ipratropium bromide and hyoscine. Knowledge of adverse drug reactions can only be developed when the prescriber has a competent comprehension of the mode of actions of drugs and their potential adverse effects.

- To improve concordance with medication, the prescriber should prescribe medication using simple regimens that require once-daily dosing whenever possible. Before adding a medicine to a medication regimen, it is important to ensure that it is not used to treat an unwanted effect of another medicine, for example, cough suppressants in a patient using ACE inhibitors such as enalapril.

- Assess the efficacy of medicines in the treatment of specific conditions. In cases where there appears to be limited benefit, substitute rather than add another medicine, for example, analgesics, drugs used to treat gastrointestinal and psychoactive agents.

- Empower patients, their relatives and families and caregivers through appropriate education in medication management. Education can take the form of an informal short teaching session supported by the provision of medication information leaflets, information details about pathological conditions and information about advisory groups.
- Frequently review the necessity of medicines, especially where the treatment may be for a limited period, for example with the prescribing of H_2 antagonists such as cimetidine and ranitidine, hyposedatives such as benzodiazepines, antidepressants such as amitriptyline, non-steroidal anti-inflammatory drugs and antipsychotics such as chlorpromazine. New medicines should be introduced only when the benefit is absolutely clear.
- Prescriptions must be legible. It is imperative that the medicines written on prescriptions should be clearly identified and the use of abbreviated forms of medicines and decimal points should be avoided.

Rational prescribing and prescribing support

Rational prescribing centres on accurately prescribing the correct medication for a pathophysiological condition, and undertaking an assessment of the efficacy of the treatment and its ability to manage the symptoms of the condition. The process of rational prescribing also focuses on the recognition of the impact of ageing and how it is necessary to titrate the dose of medicine according to the patient's needs. This means commencing treatment at the lowest strength of medicine possible, being pharmacovigilant and recognising the affects of ageing on the ability of the older person to endure the potential adverse effects of medication (Swift, 2003). Findings from recent studies highlight the need for pharmacovigilance when prescribing for the older person. Gilbert et al. (2002) reported that 37% of the prescribing problems encountered centred on the need for medication review and 18% of cases reported required additional biochemical screening. These findings highlight the need for prescribing support when making prescribing decisions. Community-based pharmacy prescribing advisors are available who can provide guidance and support when prescribing for older people.

Conclusion

Medication management is a complex concept that encompasses numerous inter-related features and is an essential feature of the NSF for Older People (DoH, 2001, 2001a). Central to this process is SAP and the use of trigger questions to develop comprehension of the degree of

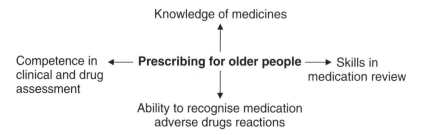

Figure 4.3 Issues central to the medication management of older people.

patient concordance with medication. Previously, pharmacists played a central role in SAP and the process of medication review with older people (Mental Health Foundation, 2001, 2004); now, with appropriate education and training, community matrons and other health care professionals undertake this role (DoH, 2005).

The medication management of patients with long-term conditions is central to the government's programme of health reforms that aim to improve the provision of health care services for older people (DOH, 2005). To achieve this goal, SAP assessors and community matrons require a working knowledge of pharmacology, experience of medication and clinical assessment and expertise in prescribing medicines to older people (see Figure 4.3).

Implications for practice

Medication management may be a relatively new term for nurses, nurse prescribers and community matrons. The key components of medication management include medication review, recognition of the adverse effects of drugs, patient education and measures to ensure that the medicines prescribed to patients continue to be effective and appropriate for the condition(s) being treated. As the number of SAP assessors increases and they take responsibility for the medication management of older patients, the care that is provided will improve as expertise develops. Now that nurse and pharmacist independent prescribers have extended prescribing roles, it is likely that they may become the next generation of SAP assessors. To accommodate this, the academic level of non-medical prescribing education and training should be commensurate with the advanced level SAP assessor programme.

Medication errors and the older person

Maggi Banning

Learning objectives

The aim of this chapter is to introduce the reader to the concept of medication errors and its role in the medication management of older people. This will centre on the following:

- an overview of the classification systems that are used to assess medication errors
- common causes of medication error
- a summary of the common forms of medication errors, such as those arising due to omissions, faults in the timing of administration, or errors that result as a consequence of self-administration of drugs by older people
- a review of errors that arise due to the supply and administration of medicines
- the prevention of medication errors and the role of the nurse or community matron in their prevention.

Introduction

Medication errors are not a new problem. According to the Medical Defence Union, 25% of the most successful claims for damages against British GPs are caused by errors in prescribing, administering and supplying medicines (Goldbeck-Wood, 1996). The medical damage to patients varied. Goldbeck-Wood found that 50% of claims involved injuries such as scarring, nerve damage or stroke; however, almost

20% of cases resulted in death, stillbirth and a termination of pregnancy. The compensation provided varied, with nearly 65% of claims settled for less than £10,000 and five claims for over £100,000 (Goldbeck-Wood 1996).

The extent of the problem

The problem of medication errors is not limited to the UK; it is a global concern. Medication errors are also costly in terms of human life, professional reputation and career and also the financial costs. So what is the extent of the problem? In the US, medication errors are the eighth leading cause of mortality with figures in the region of 98,000 people (Kester & Stoller, 2003), involving 1–2% of patients (Dean et al., 2002), and contribute to one out of 131 deaths (Koren & Haslam 1994). The annual cost of medication errors in the US is in the region of $17–29 billion (Lesar et al., 1997). Even with this high national incidence of medication errors, many US-based nurses are reluctant to report medication errors due to fears of retaliation (Pape, 2001).

In Europe, medication errors are a growing concern and a cause of consternation for health care professionals (Dobrzanski et al., 2002, National Coordinating Council for Medication Error Reporting and Prevention, 2002) and the Department of Health (DoH, 2004). Trinkle and Wu (1997) propose that medication errors contribute to the equivalent economic expenditure as in the US.

The UK perspective

Human error and need for specific education and training in prescribing practice have been strongly associated with the development of medication errors (DoH, 2004). In Building a Safer NHS for Patients, the DOH (2004) outlined the extent of the problem, illustrating the causes of medication errors, potential instigating factors and their development with regard to prescribing, dispensing and the administration of medicines. The report also examined measures and challenges related to reducing the incidence of medication error relevant to specific groups of medicines, and the impact of reducing the risk of medication errors for the National Health Service as an organisation and also for its employees. Instructions for nurses are provided with regard to the care and management of drug administration and supply.

In the UK, there are no exact figures for mortalities related to medication errors. In order to monitor the prevalence of medication errors and prescribing practice, the National Patient Safety Agency (NPSA, 2003) was introduced along with clinical governance measures (Mayor, 2001). The primary function of the NPSA is to monitor medication error rates within hospitals and provide accurate findings of the incidence in the UK. A recent NPSA report estimated that 9% of incidents were related to medicines (NPSA, 2003). Although the NPSA can provide information on drug alerts that target primary care organisations, obtaining accurate figures for medication errors is more difficult due to under reporting. In a recent drug alert, the NPSA released a statement to NHS acute trusts, primary care organisations and local health boards in an attempt to reduce medication errors related to the administration of methotrexate. The key problem related to the overadministration of the drug and the potential risk of medication error arising from its over administration as indicated by clinical groups. The NPSA provided accompanying literature in the form of a patient information leaflet highlighting the dose range and duration of administration of methotrexate (NPSA, 2004).

Dobrzanski et al. (2002) reported the incidence of medication errors provided from a small-scale study undertaken in one NHS Trust in England. Medication errors were classified according to their ability to cause serious or very serious harm to a patient or those that were potentially dangerous. Dobrzanski et al. (2002) reported the inappropriate prescribing of medical staff, which led to 578 medication errors in one NHS Trust during a period of only four weeks. This figure is unacceptably high and did not include medication errors caused by dispensing or administration error. If this figure were extrapolated, it would provide an annual estimate of 7,044 medication errors; this equates to a medication error rate of 35–70% (Dobrzanski et al., 2002). This first figure is slightly lower than the suggested medication error rate of 49% (Barber & Dean, 1998; Bruce & Wong, 2001). Although several reports illustrate the severity of medication errors in the UK, these studies tend to be small scale. Larger multi-site studies are needed to extensively explore medication errors.

The potential dangers of medication errors

Medication errors are important as such incidents could invoke a variety of problems, which range from minor discomfort, the development of drug-related side effects or an adverse reaction to a drug (Leape 1994; Bates et al., 1995). This may lead to patients having a prolonged stay in hospital (Vincent et al., 2001) or a substantial change in health status (Leape, 1994; Lesar, 1992).

Medication errors can also be a significant source of morbidity and mortality in the hospitalised patient (Hartley & Dhillon 1998; DoH, 2001b). This is particularly important as older people comprise 18% of the adult population and administer 45% of the total medicines prescribed in England (DoH, 2000–2002). Medication errors add to the spiralling costs of patient care and patient discomfort. Vincent et al.

(2001) reported that the additional costs of eight days' hospitalisation cost £290,000. However, the annual costs for treating patients for prolonged periods in hospital as a result of an adverse drug reaction to prescribed medications has been estimated to be in the region of £2 billion (DoH, 2001b). This figure does not account for patients who have been prescribed medication from health care professionals working in primary care or community settings and have developed an adverse reaction or incident due to the prescribed medication. These are unknown costs.

The spiralling costs of medical care and the impact of prolonged stay in hospital for many patients have increased interest in medication errors (Dobrzanski et al., 2002) and prompted the commitment by the NHS to reduce the incidence of serious adverse events by at least 40% by 2005 (DoH, 2001b). Interest in medication errors was partially stimulated by the Department of Health report 'An organisation with a memory' which recommended that medication errors should be reduced by 40% by the year 2005 (DoH, 2001). In Building a Safer NHS for Patients (DoH, 2004), it was recognised that medication errors that arise due to prescribing or dispensing and through the administration and supply of medicines are strongly associated with human error and lack of education. It was acknowledged that there was a need for clarity in defining potential instigating factors, and an increased awareness of measures that can be taken to reduce the incidence of medication error, such as specific education and training in prescribing practice. The challenge is to reduce the impact of medication errors caused by employees of the National Health Service and the risks of serious and potentially lethal medication errors related to specific groups of medicines. Health care employees such as nurses require assistance and instructions regarding the administration and supply of medicines and associated care for the patient.

Definitions of medication error

So what is a medication error? Numerous definitions of the medication error are available. Perhaps the most common definition is the one adopted by the NPSA (2003) and the DoH report Building a Safer NHS for Patients (DoH, 2004), that is provided by the National Coordinating Council for Medication Error Reporting and Prevention (2002) who define a medication error as 'any preventable event that may cause or lead to inappropriate medication use or patient harm while the medication is in the control of health professional, patient or consumer'.

Dean et al. (2002) suggest that:

'a clinically meaningful prescribing error occurs when, as a result of a prescribing decision or prescription writing process, there is an unin-

tentional significant reduction in the probability of treatment being timely and effective or an increase in the risk of harm when compared with generally accepted practice.' (p. 1373).

Barker and McConnell (1962), American Society for Health-System Pharmacists guidelines (ASHP, 1993), Allan and Barker (1990) and DoH (2003) produced a typology of working definitions of medication errors. These include the following:

- Omissions are errors that arise when a medication is not administered at the correct time. This frequently occurs due to staffing difficulties and occurrence of emergencies in hospitals; patients are often administered medications outside the time frame that they were supposed to be administered. This is referred to as an omission error. This excludes cases where the patient refuses the medication or instances where the patient is fasting in preparation for surgery. Omission errors can be detected by checking the patient's medication prescription chart and itemising the medications that have been omitted.
- A wrong dosage medication error occurs when the nurse or medical practitioner administers an inaccurate dose of a medicine which is within 5% of the correct strength of the prescribed medication (ASHP, 1993). This type of error may occur when the person administering the medication administers a medicine that contains the wrong number of preformed dosage units or tablets.
- An extra dose medication error occurs when the nurse or medical practitioner administers more doses of the prescribed medication than was prescribed on the patient's medication prescription chart by the prescriber. Often the additional doses of a medicine were in excess of the required dose due to misinterpretation of the prescribed order. An example of this may occur as a result of a medicine having been discontinued but not withdrawn, or where a medicine has been administered on more than one occasion when it was prescribed on a once per day basis on the prescription chart.
- The fourth type of medication error can arise when an unordered medicine has been administered to a patient. In this case the patient receives a medication that was not prescribed/authorised. In the older person the administration of unordered or unauthorised medicines can have grave consequences due to the nature of medicine interactions and the sensitivity of older people to the adverse effects of medicines.
- Wrong dosage form medication errors occur when a medicine is incorrectly written in a prescription. Medical and nurse prescribers need to be vigilant when prescribing medicines in order to prevent mistakes from occurring.

- Medication errors can occur due to the prescription being administered by the wrong route. This form of medication error will involve medicines that are administered by a route which is different from the prescribed route. For example, administering a prescription of oral valium and administering the medicine using an intramuscular route.
- The final form of medication error includes those that occur due to the wrong administration or the use of an inappropriate procedure or improper technique in the administration of a drug. This may include the splitting of medicines into two halves, in order to administer half the dose of a tablet. This form of medication error occurred following the splitting of modified release tablets, which is detrimental to the rationale underpinning this pharmaceutical preparation.

Whatever definition is accepted, medication errors are a cause for concern, particularly those that arise due to the administration and supply of medicines, as these forms directly involve nurses. Medication errors can be extremely harmful for older people due to the potential for altered pharmacokinetic and pharmacodymanic responses to drugs, therefore making medication errors is more serious in people of this age group (see Figure 5.1).

Classification of medication errors

In Building a Safer NHS for Patients (DoH, 2004), medication errors are grouped into those that do not result in harm to the patient. This includes near misses and medication errors that may be detected before they can cause any harm. This may include miscalculation of the dose of a drug that would have been prescribed to a patient, but it is corrected before administration or an error that can cause harm to the patient. An example of this form would be prescribing a non-steroidal anti-inflammatory drug for a patient with a diagnosis of gastric ulcer. This form of treatment could result in this type of patient suffering from a gastrointestinal bleed.

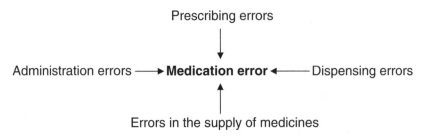

Figure 5.1   Classification of medication errors.

Medication errors have been classified in numerous ways. Lesar et al. (1997) classified medication errors as grave, very serious, moderately serious and minor. Lustig (2000) also includes errors of relatively minor significance which may be of pathophysiological significance due to their effect on the patient. Common examples included prescribing 60 mg of oral methotrexate daily instead of 15 mg weekly, failing to prescribe specific therapies such as antihypertensive medication or anticonvulsant medication, or the inappropriate prescribing of warfarin for a patient at discharge – prescribing 9 mg instead of the prescribed 3 mg (DoH, 2004).

Medication errors can also be categorised by type and then subdivided into errors occurring during prescribing or dispensing or those that occur as a consequence of the administration and supply of medicines. The categories are not always mutually exclusive; therefore, error rates for different error types cannot always be simply added to obtain an overall error rate.

One of the problems that has been encountered when defining and classifying medication errors is compounded by the fact that the most influential and significant studies that have proposed causative factors relevant to medication errors, are actually studies that were conducted in American hospitals. The main problem when attempting a direct correlation to the UK is the fact that the prescribing, dispensing and administration, and medication error reporting systems, differ from those of British hospitals (Lutener, 2001; Hartley & Dhillon, 1998). This fact should be remembered when discussing the classification of medication errors that are often reported in terms of type, quantity and whether they are caused by prescribing, dispensing or by the administration and supply of medicines within the hospital environment. However, one has to remember that medication errors are preventable; therefore, in order to assure drug safety, both safe products and safe systems are needed.

Medication errors that are caused by inappropriate prescribing, inaccurate dispensing and problems related to the administration and supply of medicines may be further examined and include a variety of associated factors (Table 5.1).

Causes of medication error

In 1991, Leape et al. systematically analysed the aetiology of adverse medication incidents and produced a classification system that permitted further exploration of the underlying causes of medication errors. This classification allowed the development of broad categories or domains which reflected the underlying problems that often result in medication errors (Leape, 1994) (Table 5.2). Leape's original work recognised that medication errors are multi-factorial and identified 26

Table 5.1 Types of medication error.

Type of medication error	Example
Prescribing	Inappropriate drug choice Calculation errors Inappropriate monitoring Therapeutic duplication
Dispensing	Calculation problems Inappropriate labelling Provision of inadequate information Confirmation bias in drug selection
Administration and supply	Drugs to the wrong patient Drugs given twice/overdose Drugs given at wrong time Drugs given by the wrong route Wrong choice of drug Drug given at the wrong rate

Table 5.2 Causes of medication error.

Causes of medication error	Exemplars
Human error	Slips and memory lapse, faulty identity checking, inadequate monitoring, staff fatigue due to workload, high error rates in medication administration due to shift work, inexperienced and inadequately trained staff. Problems associated with calculations for fluids or medicines
Technical problems	Infusion pump and parenteral delivery problems
Environmental factors	Lighting, noise, frequent interruptions
Pharmaceutical problems	Preparation errors, pharmaceutical preparation in particular injectable forms of medication
Educational problems	Lack of information about the patient Lack of knowledge of the medicine Increased number or quantity of medications per patient. Lack of effective policies and procedures
Dispensing issues	Faulty dose checking, medication services, lack of standardisation, type of distribution system used, stocks of medicines on hospital wards should be kept to a minimum
Storage concerns	Medicine stocking and delivery problems, improper drug storage
Communication problems	Faulty interaction with other services, poor communication among health care providers, failed communication. Poor handwriting which blurs the distinction between two or more medicines with similar names or that are administered by the same route or that have a similar dosage

causes which were categorised into eight themes: education, technical problems, human error, environmental, dispensing and storage of medicines, communication between staff and the pharmaceutical preparation of medicines (see Figure 5.2).

Within each category there are factors which contribute to the development of medication errors. For example, within human error there may be a memory lapse or memory slip which leads to an individual inaccurately prescribing medicines (Lesar et al., 1997; Dean et al., 2002); for example, writing 250 mg instead of 500 mg in a prescription. Memory slips are unavoidable and the DoH (2001b) states that 'human and system factors interact with the complex processes of prescribing, dispensing and administering medicines to produce an unintended and potentially harmful outcome'.

Human errors can also involve faulty checking of the patient's identity or the dose required and poor or failed communication on the administration and supply of medicines to patients. These problems can arise due to fatigue (O'Shea, 1999).

Education is an important aspect of prescribing medication. An inadequate knowledge of the patient and their condition can lead to medication errors (Lesar et al., 1997). Deficits in pharmacological knowledge can lead to prescribers writing prescriptions for medications that can be contraindicated due to the potential for adverse drug reactions, or can lead to a lack of care when titrating doses of medicines to suit the patient's requirements (DoH, 2004). For example, failing to titrate the dose of digoxin in an elderly patient suffering from renal failure; this is particularly significant as renal function reduces with age, therefore drugs such as digoxin can lead to toxicity. Deficient access to patient information, or failure to ascertain an accurate patient history, can lead to medication errors (Lesar et al., 1997; Dobrzanski,

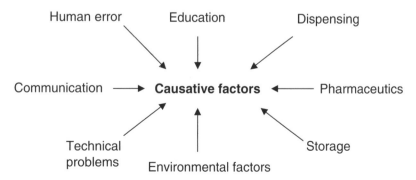

Figure 5.2 Causes attributed to medication errors.

et al., 2002) and contribute to prescribing the wrong medicines for a patient, e.g. captopril prescribed instead of capozide.

Forms of medication error

Medication errors can also arise due to the need for older people to remember complex drug regimens. This may be a problem for older people who suffer from multiple pathologies which may require treatment with a variety of different pharmacological compounds – often more than four medicines. These medicines may be prescribed more than once per day to maintain a therapeutic level, which adds to the complexity of the medication regimen. Given that many older people may suffer from impaired memory, incipient dementia or confusional states (Barat et al., 2001), this fact increases the risk of developing medication errors.

Medication errors that arise due to the supply and administration of medicines

The entry requirements for preregistration nurse education and training require that nurses are numerate. This is extremely important as the lives of patients depend on nurses who can calculate infusion rates for intravenous fluid regimens, and can convert milligrams to grams or micrograms and millilitres to litres, and read and interpret medication prescription charts. Mathematical competence is also required for nurse prescribers who write prescriptions using milligram, microgram and gram abbreviations. Nurses need to be assessed for competence as a prescriber (Banning, 2005).

Mathematical incompetence is a global concern. In the US, Pape (2001), Papastrat and Wallace (2003) and Polifroni (2002) reported that mathematical incompetence of graduate nurses led to medication errors involving patients. In the UK, nurses have been implicated in medication errors involving the incorrect administration of medicine, inaccurate drug calculations and the inappropriate use of medicine abbreviations (Bruce & Wong, 2001; Dummet, 1998; Chin, 1986; O'Shea, 1999; Hutton, 2003; Rolfe & Harper 1995). Medication errors have also been reported as a consequence of a lack of appreciation of the complexity of pharmacological regimens (Papstrat & Wallace 2003), difficulties calculating percentage dilution of fluids and drugs (Hutton, 2003), and mathematical computation (O'Shea, 1999). The importance of proficiency in mathematical computation and the need to safeguard patients against medication errors has led some countries to assess this important aspect of patient care. In Australia, pre-registration nursing students need to pass numeracy and mathematical competence assignments prior to receiving their nurse registration qualification (Manias & Bullock, 2002). Similar arrangements are used in the US, unlike the UK.

Lesar et al. (1997) found that medication miscalculations accounted for one in six medication errors. Calculation errors are not always the fault of nurses. Rolfe and Harper (1995) reported that medical doctors had extreme difficulties calculating dilution mass concentrations by conversion from percentages. In this respect, nurses can make a significant contribution by detecting medication errors in the prescriptions written by medical colleagues and supporting newly qualified housemen in the writing of prescriptions (Dobzranksi et al., 2002). But what happens when the nurse is the prescriber? Hutton (2003) found that nurse prescribers had difficulties undertaking mathematical calculations and prescribing medications accurately. It is extremely important that independent and supplementary nurse prescribers are numerate (Banning, 2005).

Factors contributing to the development of medication errors

Workload and shift work are contributory factors that can influence the development of medication errors (Lesar et al., 1997; Dean et al., 2002). Nursing is a 24-hour occupation which accommodates continuous patient care with nurses working in shift patterns of up to 12 hours. Contributory factors include the quantity of shifts worked, the type of shift work, night duty versus day duty, staffing problems (Gold et al., 1992) and the volume of patients nursed (O'Shea, 1999). However, no association has been implied between the development of medication errors and the duration of hours worked (Taunton et al., 1994; Davydov et al., 2004). These studies were fairly small scale; larger cohort, longer duration studies are needed to help differentiate associations and expand on the concept of workload and medication error.

Medication errors can also arise due the problems of using both proprietary names and brand names (Lesar, 2002; Nurse Practitioner, 2001) and also administering or prescribing medicines that have similar names (DoH, 2004). For example, prescribing frosemide (lasix) and omeprazole (losec) (Faber et al., 1991), clomifene and clomipramine (DoH, 2004) and azathioprine and azidothymidine (Landis, 1990). Errors can also arise when similar dosage strengths are presented, for example volmax 4 mg and flomax 0.4 mg (Nurse Practitioner, 2001). These forms of medication errors are common. Dean et al. (2002) identified 134 prescribing errors in one week; 34 were potentially serious. These types of errors can be accentuated when the prescriber has illegible or ambiguous handwriting (Hoffman & Proulx, 2003; DoH, 2004).

Illegible handwriting may occur in up 10% of prescriptions (Jenkins, 1993) and lead to mistakes interpreting the prescription, and dispensing errors by the pharmacist (DoH, 2004) which can be extremely harmful to the patient (Charatan, 1999).

The Guardian (1988) reported the case of a patient who spent five months in hospital recovering from the inaccurate dispensing of glibenclamide (daonil) for the treatment of a chest infection. The patient was originally prescribed amoxicillin and was left with residual memory loss. In a second case, a patient was prescribed liothyronine sodium 25 mg on discharge from hospital. The pharmacist interpreted the name of the medicine on the prescription as methotrexate 2.5 mg. The patient developed reductions in his white blood cell count and later died from an associated infection (NHS, 2002). In a third case, a patient died after receiving isosorbide mononitrate 20 mg four times per day, when the pharmacist should have dispensed felodipine four times per day (Charatan, 1999). Cases like these may appear to be extreme, but they highlight the importance of decipherable handwriting when writing prescriptions.

Dean et al. (2002) found that medication errors may occur at the time of writing the prescription and this may contribute to as much as 48% of medication errors (Ridely et al., 2004). Furthermore, incorrect prescription writing may occur when prescribers fail to adhere to the standards set and to recognised nomenclature outlined by the British National Formulary.

The nurse prescriber's role in the prevention of medication errors

As health care professionals, nurses have direct contact with patients, often on a 24-hour basis, and because of this they are in a prime position to detect and report medication errors. Nurses often serve as the final point of contact for the patient with regard to the medication use process; thus, they play an important role in risk reduction.

Errors that arise due to the different pharmaceutical preparations are common. Mistakes due to drug formulation account for 15% of medication errors (Lesar, 2002). Nurses need to familiarise themselves with the drugs that are commonly prescribed for patients in their clinical specialty; this is equally important for nurse prescribers.

The nurse prescriber's role in preventing medication errors focuses on the need to be vigilant when administering and supplying medication to patients, but also when prescribing medication independently or using protocols such as patient group directions and case management plans. Nurse prescribers should be aware of how to prevent medication errors (see Figure 5.3).

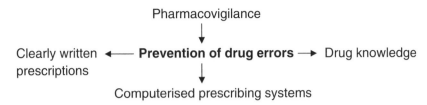

Figure 5.3 Prevention of medication errors.

Nurses can take the following precautions to prevent medication errors arising with regard to the supply and administration of medicines:

- Nurses who supply and administer medicines to patients should be familiar with the types of medicines that are commonly prescribed within their nursing specialism. This involves familiarising oneself with the dosage of the medicine, the route of administration and the typical frequency of administration, e.g. paracetamol 500 mg–1 g can be prescribed between 4 to 6 times per day, up to a maximum of 4 g.
- If new medicines are prescribed, nurses should familiarise themselves with appropriate drug information: normal dose, frequency of administration, routes of administration, potential side effects, and potential interaction with other medicines. This form of information can be found in the British National Formulary, or can be obtained from the information pharmacist, medical colleagues or the prescriber.
- In hospital settings, nurses should carefully review the patient's medication prescription charts and compare with the medications that have been dispensed, particularly when new drugs are prescribed as this is a prime opportunity for errors. Medicines should not be supplied and administered unless the name, dose and frequency of the regimen concur with what is prescribed in the British National Formulary.
- Nurses supplying and administering medicines should double-check the expiry date of medications dispensed before administering them. When there are discrepancies, the nurse should inform the pharmacy department and determine the appropriate action.
- As far as possible, medicines should be administered at the scheduled times prescribed on the patient's medication prescription chart; try to avoid missing doses, as this will interfere with maintaining a therapeutic effect.
- For medicines that are prescribed outside the normal therapeutic range or where standard drug concentrations/strengths are not available and require mathematical calculation, all calculations

should be double-checked by a second nurse, especially in cases where medicines are administered via infusion pumps.

- In cases where patients have been prescribed doses of medicines outside the normal reference range, the prescription should be verified prior to supply and administration.
- Nurses who administer medicines via administration devices such as infusion pumps should be trained in the use of such devices and comprehend the importance of administering medicines via intravenous infusion routes and the potential for side effects or the development of adverse drug reactions. It is important that nurses comprehend the mode of action of drugs that they administer, in order to assess their efficacy but also to educate the patient.
- In cases where there are two patients in a hospital ward with the same name, the medication prescription chart should provide information such as the patient's age or middle names in order to accurately identify the patient. Nurses should be vigilant in such cases to ensure that the patient's details are correctly identified prior to administering medicines. Medication errors can be prevented by ensuring that the patient is wearing the correct name band and that the details are correct.

Prescription writing education

In order to avoid errors in writing prescriptions, nurse prescribers and community matrons should review relevant medication information, in particular the need to avoid the development of side effects or adverse reactions arising due to polypharmacy, before prescribing medicines for patients. According to Dean et al. (2000), good prescribing practice is based on prescribers receiving adequate education and training in the principles of medicine dosing before they start prescribing. This approach to training can help prescribers develop skills in writing prescriptions, which in itself can improve patient safety. This is an area of practice that is not given sufficient attention in the independent nurse prescribing course, even though it is included in the curriculum of the extended and supplementary prescribing course. Numerous students on the independent nurse prescribing programme voiced their disapproval at not being provided with opportunities to practice their prescription writing skills (Banning, 2004). This is extremely important as it is a novel aspect of the nurse prescribing role and many nurses require practice in the art of accurate prescription writing.

As part of the patient consultation, nurse prescribers should also confer with the patient on their comprehension of medicines that they are prescribed, and give advice on the potential development of side effects (Kester & Stoller, 2003). Inadequate knowledge of the patient or history taking can lead to prescribing errors (Lesar et al., 1997; Dobrzanski et al., 2002). Nurse prescribers should be aware of the forms of side effects and potential predisposing factors. It is bad practice to write on prescriptions 'as directed' in terms of patient advice, as the patient may be administering more than one medication and may forget the advice that was provided at the time of writing the prescription.

Preventative measures involving prescriptions

In Building a Safer NHS for Patients, the Department of Health (2004) outlined the importance of health care professionals recognising and appreciating the variety of drug formulations that are available. It is imperative that prescribers recognise that inaccuracies in writing dosage forms can lead to medication errors, particularly when complex regimens are required (Lomaestro et al., 1992) or when prescribed medicines have unusual routes of administration, e.g. intranasal administration of Suprecur (Attilio, 1996). Care needs to be given when prescribing medicines whose mode of action is by modified release compared with medicines of a similar group that are immediate or non-controlled release, e.g. beta-adrenoceptor blockers such as atenolol (Lesar, 1992).

As mentioned previously, medication errors can arise due to incorrect calculations (Hutton, 2003). Nurses need to undertake the following:

- Be vigilant and scrutinise prescription charts for calculation or prescribing errors.
- Watch out for errors that involve prescriptions indicating that the wrong dose of a drug has been prescribed, e.g. 7.5 mg of diclofenac instead of 75 mg.
- Be careful when medicines are prescribed using decimal points. Errors can arise when the decimal point is inserted in the wrong way; diazepam .5 mg/ml instead of 5 mg/ml, or prescriptions for 5.0 mg can be mistaken for 50 mg, so it is better to write 5 mg.
- When writing prescriptions, be vigilant when writing dosage forms that include the use of decimal points, as fatal doses of medicines can be administered if the decimal point is incorrectly written on a prescription chart (Cousins & Upton, 1994). For example, avoid writing .5 ml as this can be mistaken for 5 ml; it is better practice to always include a zero in front of the decimal point e.g. 0.5 ml.
- Careful prescription writing is essential when prescribing medication doses that are less than one gram; half a gram should be written as 500 mg and not 0.5 g, and medication doses that are less than one milligram should be written as 100 µg rather than 0.1 mg.

- Avoid the use of abbreviated forms of medicines (Cousins & Upton, 1994).

Computerised prescribing systems

It is good practice for nurse prescribers and community matrons to review relevant guidelines on effective prescribing (DoH, 2000/2002, 2004) and if possible to use electronic prescribing systems to write prescriptions. Computerised prescribing systems are useful medication safety and decision support computer programmes that aim to help reduce the incidence of side effects and errors in prescribing, as they alert the prescriber to potential mistakes and can be effective prescribing tools for high-risk patients. Nurse prescribers should seek education and training in the use of these programmes in order to reduce the incidence of medication errors, and to assist prescribing practice. Nurse prescribers and community matrons should acknowledge that computerised prescribing systems are the basis of good and efficient prescribing which can enhance the individualisation of patient care (Barber et al., 2003; Barber, 2004).

In order to prevent medication errors, nurse prescribers and community matrons can undertake the following steps:

- Have regular meetings with patients to assess their medication needs.
- Regularly review patients with intricate medical pathologies that are managed using complex medication regimens (Bates, 2001; Teichman, 2001).
- Be aware of the medication errors that can arise in high-alert medicines (Zimmerman & Cousins, 2004).
- Identify risk situations and high-risk patients in order to implement appropriate prevention strategies.

Conclusion

Medication errors are potentially extremely harmful to patients, particularly older people due to their vulnerability to the toxic affects of medicines. Nurses administering and supplying medicines and nurses prescribing medicines should be aware of the prevalence, aetiology and causes of medication errors and the importance of their prevention, particularly in older people. Patient safety is of ultimate importance when administering and supplying medications or prescribing either independently, supplementarily or when using protocols. To ensure that the clinical and prescribing practice of nurses, nurse prescribers and community matrons is safe, they should receive adequate education in medicines management, including the art of writing prescriptions, and be examined in mathematical competence. Both aspects should be a compulsory component of prescriber education, especially when 45% of prescribed medicines involve older people (DoH, 2002).

Implications for practice

Nurses administering medications to older people need to be vigilant and observe medication prescription charts for potential medication errors, and if illegible handwriting is used to write prescriptions, request that the prescription be rewritten.

Nurse prescribers, pharmacists and community matrons prescribe a considerable range of medicines to patients. These medicines are used to treat a variety of conditions that range from minor illnesses to chronic diseases. As patients mature with age, the severity and number of conditions being treated often increase. This may result in the patient being prescribed more than four medicines or managed using complex regimens. This increased level of complexity can be a trigger for the development of medication errors, particularly during the writing of prescriptions. Nurse prescribers and community matrons need to be vigilant when prescribing in order to avoid unnecessary errors which may be detrimental to the health of the patient, especially if the patient is an older person.

Concordance with medication and older people

Maggi Banning

Learning objectives

The aim of this chapter is to introduce the reader to the concept of concordance with medication. In reading this chapter, the reader will gain an understanding of the following:

- the reasons why older people may be described as an 'at risk' group
- the characteristics and factors that induce an individual to become non-concordant with medication
- medication-related characteristics that can influence non-concordance with medication
- the contribution of the prescriber to improving concordance with medication through educational initiatives in the older person.

Introduction

Since the early 1990s, research into the influence of ageing on medication-taking behaviour has revealed health-belief, psychological and sociological factors that can impact on compliance with prescribed medication (Roberson, 1992). The term 'compliance' refers to taking medicines in the correct way. The term disregards the role of patients' rights with regard to taking medication and the multi-focal nature of medication-taking behaviour (Lahdenperä & Kyngäs, 2000). In contrast, the term concordance implies an equal partnership that is essential between patients and health care professionals before patients will accept the need to comply with treatment (RPSGB/Merck Sharp & Dohme, 1997). Since 1997, the term concordance has replaced compliance when referring to a patient's medication, as it is a more fitting term which embraces the patient-centred focus that is required to ensure compliance with medication (RPSGB, 1997; Mullen, 1997).

In the UK, there are 14.8 million people over the age of 65 years. This figure represents more than 18% of the population (Redfern, 1991; DoH, 2000–2002). Of the medications prescribed on an annual basis, 45% are prescribed for people of pensionable age or 65 years and over (DoH 2000–2002). This figure is exacerbated by the fact that older people have an increased tendency for physical impairment and chronic disease that require pharmacological treatment (Office of Population Censuses and Surveys, 1996).

Older people have been identified as an 'at risk' group due to the propensity to develop iatrogenic disease related to medication or chronic disease states, or as a consequence of the detrimental effects of ageing on perception, health and general well-being. This recognition led to surveillance initiatives such as the annual health check and the National Service Framework for Older People (DoH, 2001). The term 'at risk' related to the fact that many older people were considered to be socially and physically vulnerable, may suffer from pre-existing memory impairment and altered physical status, or are prone to developing adverse drug reactions from the medications they were prescribed (Walker & Wynne, 1999). One has to remember that the medication management of older people is a multi-factorial process which involves consideration of potential degeneration of physical status, increased health risks associated with increasing age and altered pharmacokinetic parameters (Hammerlein et al., 1998), and in some cases, the need to concurrently treat multiple pathologies (Grant et al., 2002). Treatment often involves the older person administering four or more medicines concurrently, also referred to as polypharmacy. Medication mismanagement can arise as a consequence of polypharmacy (Mahdy & Seymour, 1990; Lindley & Tulley, 1992; Woodhouse & Wynne, 1992). These key considerations led to the hypothesis that older people can be susceptible to medication mismanagement (Patsdaughter & Pesznecker, 1988; Winland-Brown & Valiante, 2000; Barat et al., 2001).

Difficulties in establishing a rationale

The rationale that underpins the reasons why older people are prone to mismanage their medication, and the resultant non-concordant behaviour, has been an enigma for many years. Henderson et al. (1989) and Cline et al. (1999) suggest that non-concordance with medication leads to mismanagement of medical conditions, readmission to hospital, development of adverse effects and sometimes death. Medication mismanagement in older people correlates with an increased susceptibility to develop iatrogenic disease, and adverse effects developing from prescribed medication (Mahdy & Seymour, 1990; Lindley & Tulley, 1992). Col et al. (1990) and Hill & Ball (1992) suggest that between 25% and 59% of older people fail to adhere to or are non-concordant with medication regimes. This behaviour can lead to the mismanagement of chronic disease states and increase the risk of unplanned admission to hospital. In some cases, this may be as high as 10% (Pearson et al. 2002). Despite this high figure, GPs suggest that a more realistic figure is near to 1%. This statistic relates to the failure of hospital staff to adequately prepare older people for discharge. It is suggested that medication-related unplanned admission to hospital can be prevented by improved communication between the GP and the hospital staff regarding discharge arrangements made for older people (Pearson et al., 2002).

Characteristics of the non-concordant individual

For more than two decades the characteristics of the non-concordant individual (Griffith, 1990; Davis, 1991; Barat et al., 2001) and medication-taking behaviour have been debated (Stimson, 1974; Hulka et al., 1976; Rudd, 1993; Nytanga, 1997; SCIE, 2005). Multiple reasons are proposed to explain why some older people have an increased propensity to mismanage medication (Griffith, 1990; Davis, 1991; Barat et al., 2001). Several factors contribute to medication mismanagement (see Figure 6.1).

The seminal work of Hulka et al. (1976) on medication-related behaviour examined medication-taking behaviour of patients and categorised medication error into four main forms. These included

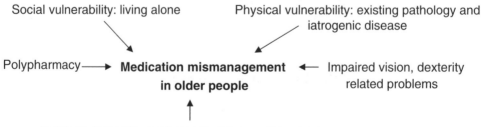

Figure 6.1 Factors related to medication mismanagement.

omissions, commissions, scheduling non-compliance and scheduling misconceptions. Omissions are lapses in taking medications and commissions are defined as administering medication outside the prescribed regimen. Both these forms are thought to be the most prevalent and directly correlated with the quantity of medicines involved or polypharmacy.

Scheduling non-compliance is defined as not adhering to the prescribed medicine regimen. Scheduling misconception forms of medication error relate to the inability to comprehend the drug regimen. These forms are thought to be a consequence of the complexities of the medication regimen imposed on the patient coupled with knowledge deficits regarding the role of prescribed medicines in the management of the pathophysiological condition. The most common contributing variables identified were polypharmacy and the complexity of regimen. This is in agreement with Allard et al. (2001) and Barat et al. (2001), who found that patient concordance with medication improved when the complexity of medication regimens was reduced (Muir et al., 2001) or when the prescription of short-acting medicines was avoided and longer-acting medications were preferentially prescribed (Rudd et al., 1992). Patient concordance with medication is also thought to improve when the prescription of unlicensed drugs is discouraged and medicines which offer the best chance of success are prescribed (Hames & Wynne, 2001).

In terms of independent factors and their relationship with medication-related behaviour, two positions are offered. Hulka et al. (1976) suggests that patient characteristics and the chronicity of the disease are independent factors that are unrelated to medication-taking behaviour. Several disease-focused studies support the view. Rich et al. (1996) and Cline et al. (1999) both reported varying levels of concordance with prescribed medication in patients with heart failure. Equivalent results were found in patients suffering from hypertension (Lahdenperä & Kyngäs, 2000), individuals with high cholesterol levels receiving medication (Applegate, 2002; Benner et al., 2002) and patients with mental health illness (Lowry, 1998). However, other studies indicate that an association exists and that the concept of non-concordant behaviour in this context is not independent of factors such as race, gender, socioeconomic status and class (Roberson, 1992; Nytanga, 1997; Boyle & Chambers, 2000). In fact, patients adapted their medication regimens according to how they were feeling, ill or healthy, implying that patient characteristics are an important aspect of non-concordant behaviour (Roberson, 1992).

Psychological theory

Psychological theories may also underpin non-compliant behaviour, and unintentional non-adherence may be more important than comprehension of the characteristics of an individual patient (Nytanga, 1997). These psychological theories include:

- the patient's individual impressions for the use of medicines will inform their ability to conform to the prescribed medication regimen
- the rationale for prescribed therapy can influence adherence to prescribed medication regimens (Mahdy & Seymour, 1990; Nytanga, 1997)
- failure to recall the regimen of prescribed medication was attributed to the conflicting advice patients received from different physicians (Col et al., 1900).

Concordance with medication is also influenced by the health beliefs of the patient. Patients need to be provided with opportunities to express their health beliefs and views on medication during the doctor–patient consultation. This process can enhance the therapeutic alliance between patient and health care practitioner (Chen, 1999) and increase the effectiveness of communication between the health care practitioner and patient, but may also involve family members and carers (Byetheway et al., 2000). The significance of patient–practitioner consultations, and the impact on the family and role of carers in relation to promoting concordance with prescribed medication, was addressed in the National Service Framework for Older People in an attempt to raise awareness of their credence (DoH, 2001). The consultation should also include discussion of factors that can impact on medication-taking behaviour which include:

- gender, race and religious influences
- patient's opinions on the rationale for the medication and duration of administration of medication – short or long term
- underpinning knowledge of the condition being treated
- patient's comprehension of the role of the medication in the management of their condition
- patient's knowledge of side effects of the individual drug.

Medication-related issues that underpin non-concordance

Polypharmacy and complicated medication regimens

Medication-taking behaviour is a multi-factorial process that may be influenced by problems such as incipient dementia, confusional states, memory impairment, impaired vision and dexerity-related problems, social vulnerability, isolation and lack of education (Banning, 2004a). All these can add to the difficulties of remembering complex medication regimens. In addition, there are problems associated with the quantity of medication prescribed, or polypharmacy, and the complexity of medication regimens. This controversial issue has been hotly debated. Rudd (1993) and Barat et al. (2001) both indicate that there is a strong correlation between polypharmacy and non-concordance with prescribed medication. This psychological theory is supported by findings that show that when the complexity of medication regimen is reduced, concordance with prescribed medication improves (Muir et al., 2001). Patients who administer complex medication regimens are prone to be non-concordant with their medication (Rudd, 1993). In most cases medicines that have a short duration of drug action need to be administered frequently, i.e. at four to six-hour intervals. This can impact on concordance, and longer acting medicines should be prescribed (Rudd, 1993). This should improve concordance with medication as it would reduce the frequency of administration of medicines and reduce the impact of polypharmacy. The simplification of the medication regimen should encourage older people to remember which drugs to take and when to take them (Rudd, 1993) and provide opportunities to regulate the time of the regimen with daily activities such as shopping and socialising (Barat et al., 2001; Muir et al., 2001).

Lack of education

As previously stated, older people are often vulnerable to the effects of medication. Pharmacovigilance, through the use of prescribing indicators, can enhance concordance with medication in older people (Challiner et al., 2003; Batty et al., 2003). Often older people have not only to come to terms and adjust socially to the detrimental effects of long-term conditions but also accept the role that medication plays in the management of their newly diagnosed condition. Part of this acceptance involves gaining an understanding not only of their condition but also the medication involved and possible medication-related side effects (RPSGB, 1996). In order to prepare older people to take responsibility for the management of their condition, it is necessary to educate them about their condition and the role of medication in its management (see Figure 6.2).

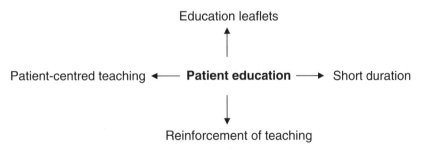

Figure 6.2 Patient education initiatives.

It is known that patients receiving treatment for the management of long-term conditions such as asthma, hypertension, high cholesterol levels or cardiac arrhythmias are often non-concordant with their medication (Lahdenpëra & Kyngäs, 2000). This increases the need for continual educational reinforcement that does not deviate dependent on the educator. Education of this kind will help the patient to understand the role of medication in the management of their condition (Lowe et al., 2000).

In hospital settings, patient education programmes should be an inclusive part of holistic patient care (Hopps, 1983; Banning, 2003). Patient education programmes should be part of the plan for discharge and should centre on the provision of appropriate medication information leaflet(s) that can help to reinforce previous teaching and promote the recall of information (Banning, 2004). It is well established that written forms of information are valued by patients (Martens, 1998) as they help patients to recall information (Banning, 2004). These initiatives should be encouraged and developed to reduce non-concordance with medication and medication mismanagement in older patients.

Following discharge, many older people mismanage their medication regimes (Wolock et al., 1987). This can lead to the development of adverse drug reactions or medication-related problems. Both these problems could easily be avoided with appropriate education (Walker & Wynne, 1999; Williams & Fitton, 1988).

Long-term educational reinforcement is an important part of the follow-on care that commences once older people are discharged from hospital. Educational reinforcement should focus on helping the patient comprehend the types of medication they are administering, especially new medications (Lowe et al., 2000), the relevance of the timing of individual doses, adherence to a complex medication regimen and instructions on the recognition of side effects (Close, 1988; Woodhouse & Wynne, 1992). Knowledge of these pharmacokinetic aspects of medication management and medication-related safety is important for the patient but also for their families and carers (DoH, 2001; Boyle & Chambers, 2000). Information of this kind can empower the patient regarding management of their illness and health-related issues (Glazer-Waldman et al., 1985) and help them make decisions about their future.

In primary care settings, patients should be encouraged to ask questions about the role of prescribed medicines in the management of long-term conditions and to express their health beliefs. Effective questioning can improve concordance as it allows patients to acknowledge the role of medication in the management of their condition (Chen, 1999), as indicated in implementing medicines-related aspects of the NSF for Older People (DoH, 2001a). During consultation with the patient, the prescriber should take time to discuss the administration of the drug, and whether the medicine can be administered with food or specific fluids. For example, tea and coffee limits the absorption of oral iron preparations such as ferrous sulphate. Similarly, grapefruit juice limits the absorption of nifedipine. Teaching patients during consultation can be an effective way to improve concordance with medication and promote patient interest in the management of their condition.

According to Cline et al. (1999), all primary care specialists should be involved in information provision and the evaluation of concordance in older people. Educating patients about their medication and potential side effects can empower patients to alter perceptions on their role in the management of their condition (Cargill, 1992).

Patient comprehension of the need to adhere to prescribed medication administration protocols

Patient comprehension of the medicines that they regularly administer plays an important role in concordance with medication, especially in the older people as they are more prone to multiple pathologies that require complex medication regimens (Lindley & Tulley, 2002). Multiple pathologies can often render the older individual physically vulnerable and impair and restrict mobility which can be influenced by the peaks and troughs of feelings of physical well-being. Coupled to this is the impact of social vulnerability, living alone, memory impairment and poor conceptualisation of the role of medicines in the management of pathological conditions, which can lead to hesitancy with respect to the renewal of repeat prescriptions. Also, relying on the goodwill of family, friends and carers to supply and administer regular medicines or collect prescriptions and medicines can have a massive impact on adherence to medication regimens. Failure to collect prescriptions on time and disrupted routines can lead to poor therapeutic effect due to omitting doses or taking medicines outside the prescribed regimen. Issues such as these can impact on concordance with medication but also increase the difficulties of trying to assess it. Although this is not a new concern, improved measures to assess poor adherence to medication regimens, medication mismanagement and the development and frequency of adverse drug reactions in the older person, are required (Rudd, 1993).

Promoting concordance with medication regimens

Concordance with medication is an extremely important aspect of medication management in the older person (Lowe et al., 2000), as non-concordant behaviour can lead to mismanagement of medical conditions and eventual deterioration of health. In order to avoid such consequences, it is important that health care professionals, nurse prescribers and community matrons relate to patients the importance of taking medicines properly and the potential detrimental affect of medication mismanagement.

Monitoring of concordance with prescribed medication can be achieved through the use of medication aids, such as drug diaries and Dosette boxes. These have been shown to improve concordance with medication (Winland-Brown & Valiante, 2000). Family members, carers and community nursing staff can help to monitor the quantity of medicines taken on a daily basis and the timings of administration. Drug diaries can be a useful reminder of the need for repeat prescriptions. Dosette boxes are beneficial for patients who have manual dexterity problems and have difficulties opening medication packaging (Atkin et al., 1994). Although the use of Dosette boxes and drug diaries have also been used to assist and improve concordance with medication, no one method has been shown to be superior (Mullen, 1997).

Patient self-medication schemes

Since the 1980s, self-medication schemes have been used as a strategy to improve patient adherence to medication regimens prior to discharge from hospital. Self-medication schemes not only increase patient's accountability for their management of their illness (Rideout et al., 1986; Kolton & Piccolo, 1988) but also help to retain patients independence (Hill & Ball, 1992). Even though patient control may increase, it has been argued that such schemes fail to improve the patient's knowledge of drugs or their concordance with medication (Proos et al., 1992; Furlong, 1996). This view may relate to the methodological issues pertinent to the study, such as patient selection and duration of study, both of which may impinge on the quality of the research outcomes. Further exploration of these schemes is needed to address the role of self-medication schemes and their contribution to medication-taking behaviour.

Information sharing between primary and secondary care settings and educational initiatives are beneficial measures that can be used to improve concordance with medication. In this respect the community matron can play a key role. Lowry (1998) and Cline et al. (1999) used negotiated planning and improved communication measures between health care professionals to increase patients' persistence with long-term medication regimens. Medication review programmes have also been used to improve concordance with medication in older people. Krska et al. (2001) reported on a pharmacist-driven pharmaceutical care planning strategy for older people based in primary care. Pharmacists undertook an in-depth medication review of older people receiving treatment for at least two chronic disorders, concurrently administering four or more medications and at risk of developing medication-related problems (Lindley & Tulley, 1992). Pharmacists attended to the patients' pharmaceutical care issues. GPs concurred with the management interventions and decisions made by pharmacists. Practice nurses were also involved in drug monitoring and reported that pharmacy interventions led to fewer older people receiving repeat prescriptions and a reduction in unplanned admission to hospital, and patient concordance with medication improved. No additional medical costs were incurred. Communication between health care professionals also improved. The benefits of this intervention outweigh any limitations. Similar interventions have proved to be successful (Goldstein et al., 1998; Mackie et al., 1999). Commitment to intervention studies such as this can enhance interprofessional working and the provision of appropriate pharmaceutical care for older people.

The prescriber's role in the augmentation of concordance with medication for older people

An important aspect of patient care is the evaluation of the patient's comprehension of their illness. Nurses and prescribers play a substantial role in the education of patients about their condition and the pharmacological and non-pharmacological management (Close, 1988). As stated earlier, opportunities for teaching are available and nurses working in both primary care and secondary care settings are in a unique position to educate patients about their medicines.

The art of teaching

Teaching is an art which develops over time and with practice. Good teaching takes time to prepare, particularly the approach used, consideration of the age of the individuals to be taught, their comprehension of the information to be transferred and how information will be reinforced. This is particularly important for older patients who have commenced new drug regimens. Teaching that is haphazard and unplanned will prevent recall of information previously provided and lead to information overload (Pullar et al., 1989). This can cause patients to become confused over the purpose of the medication and the respective regimes (Weinman, 1990).

Teaching methods used to teach older people require patient-centred approaches that utilise learning and teaching strategies which meet the individual learning needs of the patient (Walkin, 2000) and that allow time for reinforcement (Opdycke et al., 1992; Esposito, 1995). A consistent criticism of teaching programmes is the lack of individualisation; this not only negates the principles of adult learning but also the effectiveness of the programme (Cargill, 1992).

Nurses and prescribers with responsibility for teaching patients should complete the NHS Trust's approved teaching programme in order to appreciate the complexities of teaching, to gain knowledge and experience of using different approaches to teaching and to comprehend the concept of the adult learner (Knowles, 1990). By undertaking this approved course of study, nurses and prescribers can then appreciate the following:

- patients learn in different ways and no one approach will suit all learners
- patients should not be considered as one homogenous group (Knowles, 1990; Ryan & Chambers, 2000)
- where several nurses are involved in teaching the same group of patients, it is important to ensure the consistency of information that has been provided (Col et al., 1990)
- there is a need to consider how to apply teaching and learning strategies to the older adult (Tight, 1998)
- teaching should be planned so that it is structured and informative and allows time for assimilation and recall.

Teaching practicalities

It is important to ask the patient what they comprehend about their condition, and their feelings about the role of the medication in the management of the condition, especially if it is a condition that requires long-term management, such as asthma, diabetes or ischaemic heart disease. This exploration can reveal whether the patient has any concerns about the condition and its stability or the duration of treatment, or family, cultural or social concerns, and gauges the degree of acceptance of the disease and the need for pharmacological intervention. The nurse or prescriber should explore what information the patient would like to know about their respective medication(s), and their own role and the role of family members or individual carers in the management of their condition. The nurse should also consider whether family members and carers also need tuition.

The following are useful tips when preparing medication education teaching programmes:

- use diagrams to help assist discussion of key pathological conditions
- use language (avoid jargon) that the patient will understand
- teaching literature that is provided should use at least size 14 font to ensure that older people can visualise the text

- always ask the patient whether they would like family members and carers to attend teaching sessions
- for hospitalised patients, consider the need to organise teaching sessions around visiting times to allow relatives or carers opportunities to listen and ask questions
- arrange teaching sessions well in advance of the patient's discharge from hospital if possible.

Reinforcing education

Nurses, prescribers and community matrons working with patients in primary care settings will have the benefit of meeting the same groups of patients on more than one occasion. Time spent with the patient can be used to reinforce learning on the use of medicines to manage long-term conditions and the recognition of medication-related adverse side effects.

The process of teaching may appear unremittingly lengthy and time consuming; however, the benefits of gaining teaching experience through repeated practice cannot be ignored. With time, the nurse or prescriber will develop a portfolio of generic medication information that can assist future teaching sessions.

Barriers to teaching

Wagnild and Grupp (1991), in their assessment of the frequency of patient education and patient teaching prior to discharge, reported that older patients received limited education about their medicines. Four main barriers were highlighted (see Figure 6.3).

Time management and workload difficulties

Alibhai and Naglie (1999) found that only 49% of patients received education on medication. Nurse involvement in educating patients

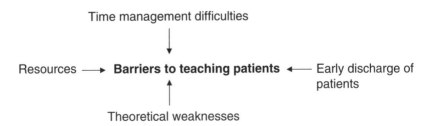

Figure 6.3 Barriers to teaching patients.

was negligible. This may reflect inadequate staffing levels, commitment to holistic patient care and patient education. Inconsistencies were found in the time health care professionals spent teaching patients, teaching styles used and the forms of information provided.

Medication education is a resource-intensive exercise that requires adequate staffing ratios, which leads to time management problems. As a consequence, nurses often provide patients' instructions about medication during the medication ward round (Webb et al., 1990) or following consultation with medical colleagues when nurses are asked to explain the significance of the consultation (Winslow, 1976). This approach to teaching is constrained by the need to differentiate patients who are willing to learn about medication matters from those who are unwilling (Syred, 1981; Corkadel & McGlashen, 1983). Such constraints can be alleviated by initiating collaborative ways of involving the ward pharmacist and medical practitioners.

The ward pharmacist can be beneficial to the education of patients and provide advice on medicines before discharge (Martens, 1998), the pharmacokinetic significance of the timing of doses, maintaining the regimen, not doubling up on tablet administration and recognising side effects (Close, 1988). This form of medication management knowledge is of relevance to both patients and their families and carers (DoH, 2001; Boyle & Chambers, 2000) as it can empower the patient about their health and its management (Glazer-Waldman et al., 1985).

Planning early discharge

The third barrier is planning difficulties associated with the early discharge of patients (Kennedy et al., 1987; Williams & Fitton, 1988). In many cases older people may be discharged early from hospital and it is up to the nurse to try to educate the patient about new medicines and new conditions. If this fails it is the responsibility of the discharge planning nurse or community matron to discuss patient concerns regarding their medication and the quantity of medicines to administer. This is particularly important for patients who have been prescribed new medicines as a replacement strategy for previous medicines, but in many cases the patient may not be aware of this and may continue to administer all prescribed medicines. Efforts should be made to ensure that patients are aware of the quantity of medicines to administer on a daily basis and the importance of having sufficient supplies of medication to manage their condition (Pullar et al., 1989). The community matron should act as the link between the hospital and primary care.

Comprehension of applied pharmacology and therapeutics

The fourth barrier that nurses and prescribers may encounter when teaching patients about their medicines is adequate comprehension of applied pharmacology and therapeutics (Latter et al., 2000). In order for nurses to be able to educate patients effectively about medicines, they themselves need to be educated in the principles of pharmacology and therapeutics (Latter et al., 2000). Deficits such as this will present problems when attempting to initiate effective patient education on medication management. For nurses who trained in the 1970s and 1980s, pharmacology education was limited in the preregistration programmes. These nurses can be proactive and request specific post-qualifying academic programmes. Gray et al. (2003) found that the nursing care of patients with schizophrenia improved when community psychiatric nurses were provided with education and training in psychopharmacology and the medication management of schizophrenia. This additional training enhanced the ability of psychiatric nurses to assess clinical compliance skills in patients. With time and the implementation of training, patient concordance with medication improved.

Conclusion

Concordance with medication is a prime concern in older people, mainly due to the potential detrimental affects of medicines. Medication mismanagement can arise due to polypharmacy, social and physical vulnerability and education deficits, and can lead to unplanned admission to hospital, adverse drug reactions and mismanagement of long-term conditions. Medication surveillance can improve medication mismanagement if used as part of a review of patient medication-taking behaviour. The benefits of hospital and community-based individualised teaching and learning strategies and pharmaceutical care planning initiatives are multiple. Nurses, prescribers and community matrons working independently and in partnership with pharmacists and medical practitioners can provide the education needed to improve concordance with medication in older people. Collaborative working practices can empower patients and also their carers to recognise the impact of medication-taking behaviour on the management of long-term conditions. Carer involvement in medication education is important, as many carers are responsible for administering medicines to older people (Bytheway et al., 2000). By undertaking these measures, one can hopefully reduce the quantity of unplanned admissions to hospital and medication mismanagement in older people.

Implications for practice

When prescribing for older people, the prescriber should consider measures that can be used to promote patient concordance with medication. These include the following:

- Longer-acting medications are preferentially prescribed in order to rationalise the quantity of prescribed medicines (Rudd et al., 1992; Allard et al., 2001).
- The use of unlicensed drugs is discouraged in favour of drugs that offer the best chance of success (Hames & Wyne, 2001).
- The use of prescribing indicators improves prescribing practice by medical practitioners and reduces the level of inappropriate prescribing (Batty et al., 2003).
- The exploration of patients' views on their prescribed medication enhances the development of a therapeutic alliance between the prescriber and the patient (Madhy & Seymour, 1990; Ryan & Chambers, 2000).
- Prescribers need to check patient comprehension of the side effects of prescribed drugs. This can act as a stimulus for additional patient medication management education (Cheek, 1997).

7

Neurophysiology, and neuropathology of ageing

Cliff Roberts

Learning objectives

This aim of this chapter is to introduce the reader to neuropharmacology and neurodegenerative diseases that commonly affect older people. In reading this chapter the reader will gain insights into the following:

- neurophysiology, neurochemistry and its relationship to cognitive function, ageing and neurodegenerative disorder
- an explanation of neurochemistry and brain function
- discussion of how early studies which were serendipitous in nature have led to an understanding of brain neurophysiology and neurochemistry
- a review of the effects of ageing on the nervous system and discussion on the pharmacological approaches used to maintain neuronal function.

Introduction

The study of brain chemistry and how neurons communicate with themselves is referred to as neurophysiology. However, when we add to this the manipulation of brain neuronal pathways and communication by drugs, we refer to this as psychopharmacology. The study of psychopharmacology has informed our understanding of the human brain, not only in terms of its microstructure but also its function in health and disorder. Depending on your own view of reductionism and the individual nature of each human being, you may or may not accept this last statement. You might consider what evidence is there to support the notion that chemicals do in fact have any effect on behaviour.

The nerve cell is a brilliant piece of biological engineering, and an understanding of its design and function is the key to brain function. Knowledge of neurophysiology is essential in order to appreciate the complexity of human behaviour.

It was not until the early twentieth century that studies provided a central dogma in functional organisation of nerve cells within the brain. There are three central tenets to this dogma. First, the neuron doctrine, which suggests that the nerve cell is the fundamental building block of the brain. Secondly, the ionic hypothesis, which encompasses the electrical nature of nerve cells in that they are capable of generating impulses that travel a considerable distance (in some cases), within a nerve cell. Lastly, the chemical theory of synaptic transmission centres on communication between nerve cells and the release of a chemical messenger (neurotransmitter), which will be recognised by a second cell. The neurotransmitter will bind to a cell surface receptor on the second cell, bringing about a change in cellular function.

In search of the nerve cell

Santiago Ramon y Cajal in 1890 managed to identify a single neurone, using silver staining. Considering that there are about a hundred billion nerve cells in the brain, this was an extraordinary feat. No one knew what a nerve cell looked like before this time, as examining the brain tissue using early lenses and microscopes revealed a literal forest of nerve cells, with no possibility of identifying an isolated nerve cell. The cell body, nucleus, axon and dendrites where identified. The synapse was inferred as a junction between one cell and another, with a very small gap between them which he called the synaptic cleft. Cajal described a principle of neurons that signals travel in one direction only, from dendrites through the cell body, axon and on to the presynaptic terminal. Additionally, he conceived the idea that nerve cells make contact with specific predetermined targets, forming predictable circuits; that is, nerve cells release their chemical transmitter onto specific targets. Cajal went on to describe sensory neurons, interneurons and motor neurons. These formed the basis of a circuit, with sensory neurons bringing information into the brain and spinal cord, interneurons being involved with processing of information, and motor neurons bringing information out from the CNS. The observations and deductions made from Cajal's studies still form the basis of neurobiology today. It is now possible to identify specific pathways and neurotransmitter systems associated with specific disease states such as Parkinson's, Alzheimer's, schizophrenia and depression, to name but a few.

Neurochemicals and synaptic communication

The point about the chemical messenger/neurotransmitter is that it is in itself a very specific messenger. In other words, the electrical message results in the release of a chemical message, which will only be received and interpreted by specific nerve circuits and certainly not by all nerve circuits. These chemical messengers are released into a cleft, which is so small it can only be seen with an electron microscope. This cleft is termed the synaptic cleft. Once the chemical has been released into the synaptic cleft it has only a very small distance to move before it will come into contact with a receptor (see Figure 7.1).

These receptors are located both on the nerve terminal from which the chemical was released and the next nerve cell membrane which lies on the other side of the cleft. For a readable overview of synaptic transmission, see Julien (1995). Some examples of neurotransmitters are acetylcholine, dopamine, serotonin and noradrenaline; more than 40 transmitters have been identified at the present time.

Synaptic communication results in information transfer. Information transfer in the brain is made up of two processes. The chemical transmitter is released into the synaptic cleft (this is referred to as the first messenger). This chemical messenger binds with its specific receptor on the post-synaptic neuronal cell membrane and brings about a biological change in the post-synaptic neuron. Intracellular processes or enzymes (referred to as the second messenger) are altered, which changes the function of the post-synaptic neuron. As this activity is occurring in the brain, examples of the change in function could be a change of mood, alteration in level of alertness or the storage of memory.

Major neurotransmitters in the brain

By far the major amino acid transmitters in the brain are γ-amino butyric acid (GABA) and glutamate. GABA is the major inhibitory neurotransmitter, whilst glutamate is the major excitatory neurotransmitter. A variety of drugs, such as benzodiazepines, barbiturates, alcohol and general anaesthetics, bind to GABA receptors in the brain and bring about a calming effect by enhancing the GABA receptors' inhibitory function. Epilepsy is thought to occur in some individuals due to an enzyme deficiency, which favours a higher concentration of glutamate to GABA, resulting in excessive excitation in an area of the brain. Glutamate is the major excitatory neurotransmitter in the brain.

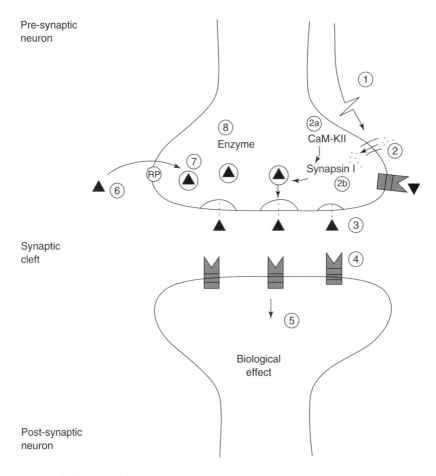

Pre-synaptic
neuron

Synaptic
cleft

Post-synaptic
neuron

1. Action potential
2. Calcium channel
2a. Calcium activates CaM-KII
2b. Phosphorylation of synapsin I → exocytosis
3. Release of neurotransmitter
4. Post-synaptic receptor
5. Biological effect
6. Reuptake of neurotransmitter
7. Repackaging of neurotransmitter
8. Degrading enzyme, e.g. monoamine oxidase (MAO) enzyme

Figure 7.1   Synaptic communication.

It acts on two different types of ionotropic receptors in the hippocampus, the AMPA receptor and the NMDA receptor. The AMPA mediates normal synaptic transmission on arrival of an action potential, whilst the NMDA receptor responds only to very rapid trains of action potentials and is involved in a process called long-term potentiation (LTP), associated with explicit memory.

The dynamic neurone, plasticity and memory

Neurones are constantly receiving and transmitting information – for example, sensory neurones are picking up information about the environment – and some of this information may be stored as memory. We all register a smell, or a visual cue or a sound that reminds us of something in the past, a memory of childhood perhaps. Repetitive training in, for example, an athlete improves psychomotor function; gymnasts, footballers, bowlers, etc. are capable of manoeuvres most of us can only dream of. Elements of their psychomotor systems are 'finely tuned'. Learning and practising complex psychomotor manoeuvres leads to changes in the strength of synaptic connections in systems responsible for these movements. Therefore the effectiveness of communication between specific cells in the neural circuits that mediate the manoeuvre is increased (Kandel, 2006). This increase in efficiency is partly brought about by an increase in the number of synapses between communicating cells, also known as sensitisation. Sensitisation is a form of plasticity, in that nerve cells are capable of changing structure and function in response to their environment.

There are also internal cellular signals, which alter cell function. An alteration in the number of these intracellular chemicals provides a communication link between receptors in the cell membrane and the internal structures of the cell. There are two types of receptor in the cell membrane, ionotropic and metabotropic. Ionotropic receptors, on binding a neurotransmitter, open or close the gate of an ion channel. Metabotropic receptors bind a neurotransmitter and activate an enzyme within the cell, for example adenylyl cyclase (AC). On activation AC amplifies the cell's response by producing a thousand molecules of cyclic adenosine mono-phosphate (cAMP). cAMP then binds to a key protein called protein kinase A (PKA). Kinases modify proteins by adding a phosphate molecule to them, a process known as phosphorylation. Phosphorylation can activate some proteins and inactivate others. In this way, phosphorylation serves as a molecular switch, turning the biochemical function of a protein on or off (see Figure 7.2). Early laboratory studies showed that in increase in cAMP strengthens the synaptic connection in glutaminergic neurons (those nerve cells releasing glutamate as a neurotransmitter), enhancing the release of glutamate.

It was also noticed that during this process the synaptic potential of the neurone was significantly slowed. Further laboratory studies identified the slow synaptic potential to be related to potassium channels. The S potassium channels close in response to rising levels of cAMP and PKA causing the slow synaptic potential, which enhances the release of glutamate. The slow synaptic potential is caused by slow repolarisation of the resting membrane potential, due to the closure of S-type potassium channels. Slowing the repolarisation stroke in the

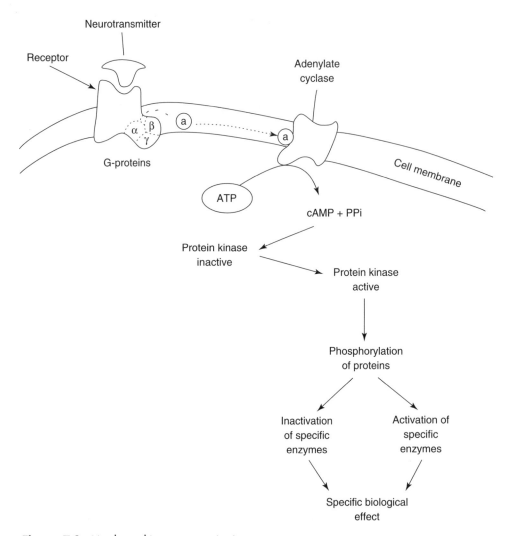

Figure 7.2 Metabotrophic receptor activation.

nerve terminal allows more time for calcium to enter the cell and calcium is essential for the release of the neurotransmitter into the synapse. These changes were identified as processes involved in short-term memory storage. The next question was how does short-term memory storage become long-term memory.

In the 1980s Jacob-Monod, Goelet and Kandel were of the opinion that long-term memory must be involved with protein regulation in the nerve cell. They also found that long-term memory requires the growth of new synaptic connections. They surmised that cytosolic chemicals must enter the nucleus and switch on genes for protein synthesis, resulting in new synaptic connections. Repeated stimulation of synapses in laboratory studies showed increasing levels of cAMP, AC and a newly discovered kinase called MAP kinase. AC and MAP kinase were observed to move into the nucleus with repeated sensitisation. Very importantly, at around the same time it was discovered that PKA, once in the nucleus, can activate a regulatory protein called cAMP response element-binding protein (CREB), which binds to a promotor sequence the cAMP response element, thereby turning on the genes that encode proteins needed for the growth of new synaptic connections. Could CREB be the key, the switch that converts short-term changes in synaptic connections to long-term changes? Continuing research in this field provided the observation that if the action of CREB in the nucleus is blocked, long-term strengthening but not short-term strengthening is prevented. Later the injection of CREB phosphorylated by PKA into the nucleus turned on the genes that produce long-term facilitation of these connections.

Following on from this, two forms of CREB were found: one that activates gene expression (CREB-1 activated by PKA), and one that suppresses gene expression (CREB-2 activated by MAP kinase). So, long-term changes in synaptic communication require both switching on and switching off of genes. But how is the new growth maintained?

Dormant mRNA molecules are found in all synapses and can become activated by an appropriate signal. A protein cytoplasmic polyadenylation element-binding protein (CPEB) is also present in all synapses and regulates local protein synthesis. CPEB is normally dormant, but is activated by serotonin. CPEB has the characteristics of a prion and when activated by serotonin it activates dormant mRNA. The activated mRNA regulates protein synthesis at the new synaptic terminal and perpetuates the memory.

We can learn a behaviour, much as discussed before about athletes. We learn how to ride a bike and once learnt we don't even think about it; we just jump on the bike and cycle. This is referred to as implicit memory. Explicit memories are those we summon up at will, or may surface following an environmental cue, or when we are reflecting on past experiences. Explicit memory involves more than one structure in the brain; there is no single 'memory area'. Explicit memory is complex and the memory which starts as 'I remember' can become very detailed, almost to the point that the memory is like watching a film or theatrical scene.

It is known that two of the areas involved in explicit memory are the hippocampus and the medial temporal lobe. Early studies involving hippocampal cells applied a very rapid train of electrical impulses to a neuronal pathway leading to the hippocampus. Connections in that pathway were strengthened for hours and in some cases days. Explicit memory involves long-term changes in synaptic communication, and this is referred to as long-term potentiation (LTP) (see Figure 7.3). LTP is dependent on a sufficient number of co-operatively active synapses working together. The increased activity persists after induction and is the neuronal basis of memory. The intensity of the rapid stimuli causes the AMPA receptor to depolarise the cell membrane. This depolarisation results in an ion channel in the NMDA receptor opening, allowing calcium to flow into the cell. The influx of calcium acts as a second messenger, triggering LTP. It is also thought to involve changes in gene expression and insertion of AMPA glutamate receptors on post-synaptic membranes (Malinow & Malenka 2002) within the network. This increases the efficacy of communication within the network and it is long lasting. It is therefore not surprising that with age there is a decline in these processes, i.e. gene expression involving the production of AMPA receptors through protein synthesis (Guzowski et al. 2000; Jones et al. 2001).

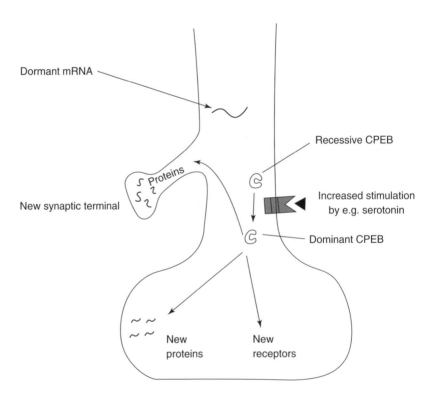

Figure 7.3 Proposed mechanisms in long-term potentiation. New proteins are involved in the growth of new synapses. New receptors will also be produced both pre- and post-synaptically (a theoretical model). Repetitive stimulation results in long-term structural changes.

Changes in neuronal activity and communication in the ageing brain

The options for neuronal changes in the ageing brain include loss of neurones, loss of synaptic connections, a reduction of neurotransmitter release into the synapse or loss of receptors on the post-synaptic cell membrane. Some neurons in the brain may have up to 40,000 synaptic connections, i.e. one neurone may receive 40,000 incoming messages from other neurones. These connections develop during foetal life and continue to form after birth. The process of growth in terms of these connections is termed dendritic arborisation and in a healthy young brain these structures contribute a significant amount to total brain growth (plasticity), bulk and weight. These mechanisms are thought to support cognition, and some of these processes are affected during normal ageing. Notably, cognitive functions that rely on the medial temporal lobe and prefrontal cortex, such as learning, memory and executive function, show considerable age-related decline (Burke & Barnes 2006). In middle age and as a natural process of ageing, dendritic arborisation slows down and connections begin to reduce in number.

Historically it was suggested that age-related reductions in brain weight were mostly due to a decline in neuronal number in all cortical areas (Brody 1955). More recently it is suggested that small region-specific changes in dendritic branching and spine density are more characteristic of the effects of ageing on neuronal morphology (Uemura 1985; Markham et al., 2005).

A fundamental function of neurones is that of communication; the chemical aspects have been discussed above. However, the electrical properties of neurones essential for communication mean that they have a resting membrane potential (RMP), and a threshold value that must be reached before an action potential (AP) can be elicited. A wave of depolarisation, i.e. a change in polarity, is followed by a wave of repolarisation and hyperpolarisation. Two things to bear in mind when looking at this are:

- neuronal cells are excitable and if the RMP reaches threshold there will be an action potential, the end result of which will be the release of the neurotransmitter from the nerve terminal
- when a neurone is hyperpolarised, i.e. the resting membrane is reset to a more negative value, it becomes more difficult to excite the neurone because more stimulation is required to move the RMP to the threshold value, and elicit an AP.

With age there are changes in calcium (Ca^{2+}), homeostasis (Toescu et al., 2004), which results in two pathological problems:

- Plasticity deficits, i.e. disruption to growth and morphology of neurones (Foster & Norris 1997).
- The change in Ca^{2+} homeostasis results in an increase in outward potassium (K^+) currents. This removes cations (K^+) from the interior of the cell, resulting in an increase in hyperpolarisation (Landfield 1988).

What causes cellular damage with ageing?

Oxygen free radicals and the free radical theory

Oxygen free radicals represent the most likely contender to explain a mechanism which might underlie the ageing process. All aerobic organisms produce free radicals, predominantly superoxides, formed during the reduction of molecular oxygen (Zhu et al., 2004); that is, these superoxide free radicals are produced when glucose in the presence of oxygen is metabolised in the mitochondria. These superoxides are also referred to as reactive oxygen species (ROS) and are thought to have a deleterious effect on cells. This increase in oxidation and the production of reactive oxygen species is termed 'oxidative stress'. The production of superoxides during oxidative stress is speculated to be pathologically important in neurodegenerative diseases such as Alzheimer's and Parkinson's (Smith et al., 1995; Cross et al., 1987). Oxidative stress is thought to produce pathological changes in all classes of biomacromolecules, i.e. DNA and RNA, proteins, lipids and sugars. There is increasing evidence that oxidative stress is involved with the very earliest neuronal and pathological changes characteristic of neurodegenerative diseases, and that these changes result in deterioration in neuronal function and communication, for example, Alzheimer's disease and Parkinson's diseases.

It is important to bear in mind that whilst the free radical theory is useful, it remains unproven. Questions remain to be answered such as, are oxygen free radicals causative or merely correlated with ageing (Burke & Barnes, 2006)?

Neuropathology of Alzheimer's disease

The neuropathological findings of Alzheimer's disease (AD) brain tissue is characterised by the presence of intracellular neurofibrillary tangles (NFTs) and senile plaques (SP), with a core of amyloid beta-peptide (Aβ) (Sultana et al., 2006). The NFTs are composed of hyperphosphorylated tau and neurofilament proteins. These proteins are important components of the neuronal cytoskeleton (Reddy & McWeeney 2006). The SP are extracellular and consist of a core of Aβ, which is derived from amyloid precursor protein (APP) (Rutten et al.,

2005). These senile plaques are found at the centre of an area of dystrophic neuritis, which is coupled with synaptic loss. The neuronal cytoskeleton and microtubule structures become significantly destabilised. This leads to disruption of vital cellular functions such as neuronal transport and loss of cell shape, resulting in degeneration of the affected brain areas (Mandelkow et al., 2003; Stamer et al., 2002). As a consequence, the predominant affects are reduction in cholinergic transmission and other neurotransmitters.

The nuclei of the hippocampus are closely involved in memory and processing (Braak & Braak 1997). As described above, oxidative stress is thought to produce pathological changes in all classes of bio macromolecules, i.e. DNA and RNA, proteins, lipids and sugars. AD may arise as a result of protein oxidation, lipid peroxidation, DNA oxidation, glycation end products, and ROS formation. Oxidation certainly causes deleterious changes in metabolism in all of these macromolecular groups. A prime candidate for the neurodegeneration seen in AD brain is protein oxidation. Proteins modified by oxidation are those involved in pathways of energy metabolism, excitotoxicity, proteosomal dysfunction, phospholipid asymmetry, cholinergic dysfunction, and neuritic abnormalities consistent with pathological alterations found in AD brain and loss of function (Castegna et al., 2004; Hensley et al., 1995; Sultana & Butterfield, 2004); thus providing a potentially unfavourable association between oxidation, protein metabolism and neurodegeneration found in the AD brain.

Evidence also suggests that abnormalities in calcium homeostasis, inflammatory changes and elevated cholesterol may play a pathogenic role in AD (LaFerla, 2006).

Pharmacological strategies

In AD, nerve cell loss occurs principally in the nucleus basalis of Meynert. The degree of memory impairment correlates closely with the loss of cholinergic transmission in the temporal lobe and other cortical regions (Coyle et al., 1983). The main pharmacological strategy in AD is to improve memory and if possible slow the progression of the neuropathology and therefore the symptoms. Numerous proprietary pharmacological products are currently being developed, but only a few are being studied for prevention of AD. Randomised clinical trial data are available for agents such as calcium channel blockers, angiotensin-converting enzyme inhibitors, pravastatin, simvastatin, conjugated oestrogen, raloxifene, rofecoxib, AMPA agonists and cholinesterase inhibitors, regarding efficacy for Alzheimer's disease prevention. At least four large prevention trials of conjugated oestrogen, selenium and vitamin E, Ginkgo biloba and statins are currently underway (Doraiswamy & Xiong, 2006). Cholinesterase inhibitors (ChEIs), remain the main group of drugs used in the treatment of symptoms (Sabbagh et al., 2006). The most commonly prescribed drugs for AD are cholino-mimetic drugs, such as donepazil, rivastigmine and galantamine. These drugs can be used in the treatment of mild to moderate AD, but currently are only licensed in the UK for the moderate stage of the disease. Evidence from AD sufferers in the early stage of the disease is that there is an improvement in memory and quality of life. However, these drugs are not prescribed in the early stages as the National Institute for Health and Clinical Excellence (NICE) only supports their use once the moderate stage is reached. This position remains at the present time a highly contentious issue. There is also contention over whether these drugs modify the disease process and delay cognitive and functional progression of AD pathology or improve symptoms with no effects on the course of AD pathology. Time will be a factor in establishing their potential in disease modification.

Cholinergic therapy is targeted at a cortical cholinergic deficit, which in itself arises during normal ageing. Two-thirds of all humans have cortical Aβ deposits at the age of 70, increasing to 90% by the age of 90 (Davies et al., 1988). Cortical Aβ deposits in non-demented ageing humans are associated with a more pronounced cholinergic deficit relative to those lacking or having few Aβ deposits (Katzman et al., 1988; Porter et al., 2004).

It is suggested that cortical cholinergic deafferentation may be the cause of age-related Aβ deposition (Beach et al., 2000). Animal studies have shown that rats with lesions in the nucleus basalis magnocellularis (NBM) have elevated levels of Aβ (the NBM supplies the cerebral cortex with its cholinergic innervation).

There is considerable preclinical, radiologic and clinical evidence that cholinergic drugs such as ChEIs may be disease modifying. The linkage of cholinergic receptor activation to βAPP processing suggests that cholinergic pharmacotherapy may influence amyloid deposition, a fundamental process thought to underlie disease progression (Sabbagh et. al., 2006).

Side effects of these drugs are related to increased synaptic cholinergic activity, due to the mechanism of action of ChEIs, i.e. the inhibition of the enzyme AchE, which results in an increase in the concentration of acetylecholine in the synapse in all cholinergic systems. Few clinically significant drug–drug interactions with ChEIs have been identified. The most common adverse effects, related to cholinergic stimulation in the brain and peripheral tissues, include gastrointestinal, cardiorespiratory, extrapyramidal, genitourinary and musculoskeletal symptoms, as well as sleep disturbances. There is debate as to the severity and cause of side effects experienced by patients, resulting in discontinuation of the drug and continued poor quality of life, for both sufferer and carer. It is reported that gastrointestinal side effects are common, but this data is from clinical trials where a side effect is reported regardless of its ferquency and severity (Keren, 2005). Also, dosages in clinical trials are enforced, whereas in clinical practice physicians can reduce the impact of side effects through slower titration and dose adjustments tailored to the individual.

Neuropathology of Parkinson's disease

Parkinson's disease (PD) is a neurodegenerative disease of unknown cause. Age is the single most consistent risk factor, and with the increasing age of the general population this disease will undoubtedly continue to rise in the future.

The major signs of PD are tremor, rigidity and akinesia. Pathological findings are characteristic, progressive death of selected populations of neurons. These include the dopaminergic neurons of the pars compacta of the substantia nigra, selected aminergic brain stem nuclei (catacholaminergic and serotonergic), the cholinergic nucleus basalis of Meynert, hypothalamic neurons, and small cortical neurons mainly in the cingulated gyrus, entorhinal cortex, olfactory bulb and autonomic neurons in the gut.

There is a regional loss of striatal dopamine in the dorsal and intermediate subdivisions of the putamen. These changes are not seen in normal ageing and this loss is thought to account for the akinesia and rigidity. Dopamine deficiency in the nigrostriatal pathway accounts for most of the clinical motor features of PD. Within the above regions and especially in the dorsal motor nucleus of the vagus are found another pathological feature, namely that of degenerating neuronal processes or Lewy neurites. The Lewy body is an eosinophilic hyaline inclusion with a targetoid appearance. The accumulations of neurofilaments within the Lewy body are thought to be chiefly due to post-translational changes following normal syntheses of these proteins. The mechanism of Lewy body formation remains uncertain. However, the changes may arise from toxic processes in the cell resulting in protein aggregation, and may therefore interfere with structural functions of neurofilaments in axons, resulting in dying back of the axonal connections from the pars compacta of the substantia nigra to the striatum. Mutations in single genes have been shown to cause PD; however, these only account for a small number of cases. Alpha-synuclein is abundant in presynaptic terminals, Lewy bodies and in neuronal inclusions found in diverse neurodegenerative disorders such as PD, diffuse Lewy body disease and the Lewy body variant of AD. The Lewy bodies are thought to alter structural functions of neurofilaments in axons. Accordingly, this is thought to result in loss of axonal connections from the pars compacta of the substantia nigra to the striatum.

There is a body of evidence suggesting PD pathology results from an excess of reactive oxygen species, increased levels of iron and increased oxidative stress. This pathology most likely arises from mitochondrial dysfunction and altered oxidative metabolism. The resulting energy failure of the cells involved could leave the cell susceptible to apoptosis. The heightened and prolonged oxidative stress may arise from toxic by-products of dopamine metabolism. Excitotoxicity results in persistent activation of glutamatergic receptors, increases intracellular levels of calcium and results in the release of iron from ferritin, lipid peroxidation is induced and impairs mitochondrial function. This explanation of a potential mechanism in PD pathology is supported by the finding that cells containing the calcium-binding protein calbindin are selectively preserved in PD. It is also observed that neurotrophic factors such as Glial-derived neurotrophic factor and brain-derived neurotrophic factors are protective and confer the ability to regenerate nerve processes in dopaminergic neurons. In PD there may be a dysfunction in the production or release of these factors, resulting in degeneration of dopaminergic cells.

It is suggested that cognitive dysfunction is associated with the degree of medial nigral cell loss and involvement of projections to the caudate nucleus. In post-mortem examinations, Hughes et al. (1993) found that 44% of patients with PD had dementia in life and of these 29% had coexisting AD, 10% had cortical Lewy bodies and 6% had a vascular cause, leaving 55% with no identifiable cause of dementia other than Parkinson's disease.

Pharmacological approach in the treatment of PD

As apoptosis in dopaminergic neurons is the major finding in PD, drugs aimed at enhancing dopaminergic transmission are the mainstay in the pharmacological treatment of the disease. Some controversy exists over this approach, as enhancing dopaminergic transmission may result in excitotoxic metabolism as described above, although there are no clinical or experimental data to support this hypothesis. However, there is evidence that delaying therapy with levadopa until pronounced symptoms are present results in motor complications developing more rapidly than in patients treated earlier in the course of their illness (Lang & Lozano 1998).

Levadopa continues to be the most effective pharmacological agent in the treatment of PD at the present time. The optimum therapeutic effect of Levadopa is maintained for around five to seven years, depending on the stage of PD on initial prescription. Underlying pathological disease progression will ultimately result in an increase of the severity of symptoms. Life expectancy is increased, with survival significantly reduced if administration of the drug is delayed.

Anticholinergic agents (e.g. benztropine), amantadine (NMDA antagonist) and selegiline (monoamine oxidase B inhibitor) can provide mild to moderate beneficial effects in the short term, and delay the introduction of levadopa by around 9 months. Levadopa and dopa-

mine agonists will then be required to reverse deterioration of muscular co-ordination.

It is important to review the mechanism of action of these groups of
drugs in order to explore the pharmacodynamic principles of therapeutic effect and side effects.

Conclusion

This chapter set out to examine the basics of neurophysiology and
pharmacology necessary to understand the pharmacodynamic principles of mechanism of action, therapeutic effect and side effects of drugs
used in the treatment of AD and PD. A sound understanding of synaptic communication will enable the reader to grasp the principles of
pharmacology pertinent to pharmacotherapy. The pathophysiology of
these neurodegenerative diseases has been explored in relation to age
and onset of symptoms.

Implications for practice

- Clinical trials, along with qualitative evidence from sufferers of these
  neurodegenerative diseases, will improve the efficacy of pharmacological
  intervention and therefore quality of life.
- A working knowledge of pharmacology will enable the health care worker
  to provide efficacious care and support to this end.
- In order to efficiently manage older people with long-term conditions such
  as Alzhiemer's disease and Parkinson's disease, nurse prescribers and
  community matrons need to have a working knowledge of neurophysiology, neuropathophysiology and recent advances in relevant applied pharmacology and therapeutics.

The management of the older person with a long-term condition

Maggi Banning

Learning objectives

This chapter will focus on the management of long-term conditions, also referred to as chronic disease management. This will be achieved using the following objectives:

- to critically examine the Government's policy on the management of people with long-term conditions
- to assess the role and contribution of the National Service Frameworks in the management of people with long-term neurological conditions
- to investigate the potential impact of the NHS Improvement Plan (DoH, 2004c)
- to critically analyse the education and training and professional responsibilities of the community matron in the management of people with long-term conditions
- to explore the role of the carer/lay carer in the medication management of the older person
- to propose the future direction of the medication management of older people.

Introduction

There are 17.5 million people in England who receive treatment for the management of a long-term condition (DoH, 2004c, 2005c). This accounts for 60% of the population of England. Of these, 6.8 million people are unable to cope with the day-to-day management of their lives (DoH, 2004b). The management of older people with long-term conditions has a huge impact on GP's practices and accounts for 81.6% of GP consultations (DoH, 2005). Medication plays a crucial role in the management of long-term illness. Many older people are prescribed six or more medications. The daily administration of this quantity of medicines increases the risk of medication mismanagement, through either the development of medication errors or adverse reactions to drugs (Mannesse et al., 1997). Adverse drugs reactions may arise due to the polypharmacy but also by poor adherence to the prescriber's instructions (Ellenbecker, 2004). Polypharmacy and the effects of ageing also increase the risk of sensitivity to the pharmacodynamic and pharmacokinetic effects of drugs (Shelton, 2000).

The current government are committed to using the skills, experience, knowledge and motivation of non-medical health care professionals to improve the health care services that are provided to older people. A plethora of documents has been generated that focus on the modernisation of the NHS; these include the National Service Framework for Older People (DoH, 2001), the National Service Framework for Older People: Medicines and Older People (DoH, 2001a), the NSF for Long Term Conditions (DoH, 2005), Supporting people with long term conditions; An NHS and Social Care model for improving care for people with long-term conditions (DoH, 2005b), the extension of nurse and pharmacist prescribing powers (DoH, 2006), Our Health, Our Care, Your Say (DoH, 2006a) and the more recent A new ambition for old age: Next steps in implementing the national service framework (DoH, 2006c). The creation of the community matron role has been influential in the development and implementation of an agenda to transform the manner in which health and social care services are provided.

Government policy and long-term conditions

In supporting people with long-term conditions: An NHS and Social Care model for improving care for people with long-term conditions (DoH, 2005b), the government illustrate how it expects to support people to live with long-term conditions, by improving their quality of life, by reducing the incidence of unplanned admission to hospital and through the prevention of premature death. It is estimated that 75% of people over the age of 75 years who are managed for long-term conditions will benefit from the projected plans.

The NSF for Long Term Conditions (DoH, 2005) outlines several key themes that aim to improve the quality of life of older people and those with long-term illness. These include the following:

- joint working across all disciplines
- promotion of independent living
- easier and timely access to services
- integration and use of multi-disciplinary teams
- care planned around the needs and choices of individuals
- integrating specialist and generalist advice in addition to cross boundary working
- provision of care in the least intensive setting and the minimisation of unnecessary visits and admissions.

Supporting people with long-term illness is viewed as a national health priority and one that can be achieved through the provision of individualised care. National targets include reducing the quantity of unplanned admission to hospital in the older people age group by 5% by 2008 and increasing the proportion of people supported to live in their own home by 2007/2008. These targets are primary care driven and can be achieved though the development of individualised care plans that involve both case finding and case management criteria (Figure 8.1).

Philp (DoH, 2006c) outlines the next stages in the development of the NSF for Older People. Attention is drawn to the problems of providing an integrated service for older people, as illustrated in DoH (2005b). Targets set by the framework are not being fully met and the care that is provided is often patchy, with mismatches between the needs of the older person and the care that is actually provided. It is estimated that 25% of acute trusts are not contributing to a co-ordinated multi-professional falls service. Furthermore, in some cases older people who are hospital inpatients do not receive a comprehensive specialist assessment or the planning that is needed to ensure their safe return to their homes. Even though procedures for supported discharge planning may be in place, communication between hospitals and the community can be patchy leading to disjointed planning and inadequate provision of care following discharge from hospital (Morris et al., 2006).

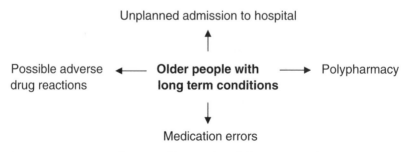

Figure 8.1 Factors influencing older people with long-term conditions.

Phelp (DoH, 2006c) highlights the need for new protocols to manage emergency responses to crises caused by common problems such as falls, stroke, transient ischaemic attack, fall or delirium. Older people with acute medical conditions accompanied by mental health problems such as depression or dementia are often nursed in care homes or hospitals where the care they receive is insensitive, and the provision of specialist psychiatric support is limited (Sampson et al., 2006). Overt age discrimination, albeit uncommon, may be associated with problems such as negative attitudes to older people. This problem needs to be tackled. With the implementation of a target of a new ambition for older people: Next steps in implementing the national health service framework (DoH, 2006c), it is for each NHS provider to identify an individual who is responsible for protecting and promoting the dignity of older people.

An additional target is proposed with respect to older people newly diagnosed with stroke. Each patient with a new history of stroke should have an appointment to be seen by a neurovascular physician within one week of diagnosis. Older people should not be denied specialist, multi-disciplinary assessment and care even when rehabilitation units may be closed or when specialist services are limited (British Geriatrics Society, 2004; Barrett, 2005; Morris et al., 2006).

Improvements in care co-ordination between the NHS and local authority services and hospitals can be implemented through practice-based commissioning. This will allow greater consideration of the policies involving health care professionals, such as GPs and the new GMS contract and the physical, financial or social parameters for managing long-term conditions.

The NHS Improvement Plan

The NHS Improvement Plan was implemented in 2004. The key goals of the plan (DoH, 2004c) were to deliver a better NHS service underpinned by the provision of high quality personalised care that meets the expectations of individuals and empowers them by offering choice. This plan aimed to reduce the waiting times for NHS services and, in doing so, transform the NHS from a sickness service to a health service. Tackling inequalities in health and concentrating on the provision of care to individuals with long-term illnesses such as asthma, diabetes or heart disease could improve service provision.

The Expert Patients Programme was designed to empower patients to manage their own health care through the provision of expert clinical support and advice by specialist GPs and other health care professionals. The Improvement Plan aimed to ensure a series of illness prevention measures to support people to improve their health, for example tackling obesity and cigarette smoking. In hospital settings,

NHS Foundation hospitals will offer patients choice of care facilities through the use of independent sector providers. Likewise, in primary care, commissioning of services to independent sector organisations will be encouraged. These developments will be facilitated by the development of more diverse roles such as the community matron and by the use of specialist GPs.

Implementing the NHS Improvement Plan (DoH, 2005) illustrates how the Improvement Plan has been executed and the benefits that patients have received following its implementation, particularly in the management of long-term conditions.

The evolvement of the community matron

As discussed in Chapter 1, the development and implementation of the community matron's role was one which aimed to make best use of nurses' skills and experience, and makes use of their abilities to effectively manage patients and is central to their case management initiative (DoH, 2004c, 2005a, b). For the government, the development of this advanced role focuses on skills and professional competence commensurate with those identified in the knowledge and skills framework. By acting as an advanced practitioner, it is hoped that the community matron will work autonomously and act as a link between primary, secondary and tertiary care settings by providing clinical management and person-centred care for older people suffering from multiple long-term conditions, accompanied by care co-ordination (DoH, 2005d). Key goals of the community matron role included:

- to reduce the number of emergency beds occupied by older people by at least 5% by 2008 (DoH, 2005b)
- to integrate all elements of care, and allow patients to function better and improve their quality of life
- to increase choice for patients and enable them to remain in their homes and communities
- to help patients, their carers and their families to plan for the future.

The community matron is an extensive role that was implemented in 2005 (DoH, 2005). The role is multi-functional and aims to offer the least intensive care in the least intensive setting with a focus on patients in the community, where the highest burden of patients exists. The role aims to build partnerships with secondary care physicians, social service professionals and GPs, with an aim of identifying patients who are thought to be vulnerable due to having two or more unplanned admissions to hospital in the last six months, having pre-existing co-morbidities and concurrently administering four or more medicines. Individuals in this high-risk category require the care of a community matron who can develop an individualised plan of care with the patient, their carers and families that is based on their medical, nursing and social care needs and that offers the patient choice.

The community matron role is commiserate with the advanced level practitioner as it encompasses 50 competences, which include case management of 50 people with long-term conditions, physical assessment skills, diagnostic reasoning, supplementary prescribing for specialist conditions, repeat prescribing, therapeutic drug monitoring and the recognition of side effects or the adverse effects of drugs (DoH, 2005d). For many community nurses, in particular district nurses, this new area of practice may be viewed as an extension to their role in the management of patients with long-term conditions; however, for senior nurses who predominantly have developed their knowledge, skills and experience in secondary care settings, the role of the community matron will be a new venture. Advice is available for senior nurses making the transition from single care environments such as hospitals to community settings (DoH, 2005d).

The education and training of the community matron

The education and training scheme aims to redesign the nursing workforce in order to prepare nurses for advanced clinical roles; this is commensurate with the Agenda for Change, Knowledge and Skills Framework. Nurses who complete all stages of the education and training scheme will be referred to as advanced level practitioners, as indicated by the NMC (DoH, 2006b). This intense education and training programme aims to provide community matrons with the knowledge and skills to undertake advanced level practice that will enable them to provide the physical, mental health and social care needs for patients with intense and complex needs.

The education and training of community matrons was developed from the community matron and case manager pilot educational programme (DoH, 2005d). The programme focuses on nine domains. Although all domains are taught at Master's level, community matrons are not expected to study for a Master's degree; it is expected that some senior nurses already possess postgraduate qualifications. The domains include the following:

- *Leading complex care co-ordination.* Teaching on this domain involves providing community matrons with an in-depth knowledge of issues such as health and well-being related to people with long-term conditions, comprehension of government policy and guidance on long-term conditions, communication, legislation and ethical concerns related to the management of people with long-term conditions. Teaching also involves ensuring that the community matron is competent in the assembly, organisation and co-ordination of complex care packages that support the effective and efficient delivery of high quality personalised care plans.

- *The principles of advanced clinical practice.* This domain focuses on the preparation of the community matron to work autonomously and efficiently, and show competence in the ability to assess and perform diagnostic tests that allow the production of a differential diagnosis and prescribe medication. These advanced practice procedures centre on the ability to undertake a physical assessment of the patient, accurately prescribe and interpret diagnostic tests and undertake both extended and non-medical prescribing relevant to the management of long-term conditions; in addition, to demonstrate competence in clinical reasoning, client-centred decision-making, and managing cognitive impairment and mental health well-being. In order to achieve these goals, the community matron will be educated in the principles of applied pharmacology and therapeutics, systems-based pathophysiology, prognosis, medicines management, differential diagnosis of long-term conditions, inter-personal psychology and communication theory.

- *Proactively managing complex long-term conditions.* Teaching of this domain centres on comprehending the impact of socio-economic and personal factors and lifestyle choices on people with long-term conditions. Teaching will also focus on undertaking a risk assessment, educating patients, and comprehension of the support mechanisms that are needed to care for people in their home environment. Teaching also focuses on the development of skills in making informed choices about the care offered to older people with long-term conditions and making decisions about the management of individuals with complex needs.

- *Managing cognitive impairment and mental well-being.* This important domain focuses on developing community matron skills in the assessment of mental health and recognition of potential deterioration in mental health status, and need to refer for specialist management. It is expected that this important domain is integral to all domains. Community matrons will be taught the basic principles of mental health status – physical, behavioural, emotional and psychological indicators – in addition to theoretical instruction on the recognition of depression, diversity, discrimination and stigmatisation, use of therapeutic interventions and advanced interpersonal psychology.

- *Supporting self-care, self management and enabling independence.* The aim of this domain is to ensure that the community matron is theorised in the importance of prompting independence, maintaining the patient's dignity and maximising choice for patients. This will be achieved through improved comprehension of the cognitive behaviour techniques, impact of long-term conditions and lifestyle choices on daily living and skills in self-advocacy, individual rights, conflict and dispute management, teaching, empowering, enabling, coaching, learning and working in partnership with patients and carers.

- *Professional practice and leadership.* The focus of this domain is to prepare community matrons for leadership roles. These roles involve making decisions, taking the lead and facilitating service improvements, and possessing the clinical credibility to provide effective leadership that supports improved clinical practice. To achieve these skills, community matrons will be taught the principles of advanced leadership, professional accountability, workforce and professional development, supervision and appraisal, reflective practice, change management and organisational development and issues central to professional and personal competence.
- *Identifying high-risk patients, promoting health and preventing illness.* The topic of this domain is the health education and health promotion needs of the very high intensity user. The community matron will receive education and training in the social construction of health and illness, evaluation methodologies and associated ethics, how to manage people's health and prevent further deterioration of long-term conditions and skills in how to interpret and analyse public health data.
- *Managing care at the end of life.* This domain features on developing knowledge and understanding of how individuals respond to stress, the changes and losses associated with life stages, and the assessment and planning strategies that are offered to patients and their families with respect to the terminal care needs of patients. Emphasis is placed on the importance of choice in relation to terminal care and skills associated with dying and bereavement.
- *Interagency and partnership working.* This final domain focuses on the education and training and role preparation to ensure that the community matron comprehends the concept of collaborative and interagency working and develops competence to work collaboratively with professionals and stakeholders across organisational and professional boundaries in order to provide efficient personalised care; and can provide leadership in facilitating service improvement to individuals under their care in addition to developing advanced skills that allow the community matron to communicate proficiently with individuals and to manage conflict and dispute.

It is recognised that many community matrons may be experienced nurses in a given speciality. The recognition of prior learning is important and self-assessment tools should be available to permit experienced nurses to identify gaps in their knowledge and skills; this can be an intrinsic motivator for students. A predominant feature of the educational programme is work-based learning. Employers have to be committed to developing senior nurses for this role and must be available to provide both workplace mentorship and supervision that will provide the necessary theoretical and practical education and training. This can be facilitated through protected time and providing opportunities for coaching, mentoring and inter-professional learning. Supervision and mentorship may be provided by GPs, geriatricians or nurse practitioners. Core competencies are extracted from the Agenda for Change, Knowledge and Skills Framework that are sufficiently generic and non-discipline specific to promote inter-professional learning activities to be developed. Mentoring and supervision should be based on the attainment of theoretical and practical skills in medical assessment, history-taking skills, and aspects of chronic disease, mental health and the ageing process. The success of work-based learning focuses on the creation of a learning environment that actively promotes learning and increases the confidence of individuals, but also permits access to specialist mentors who can assist the development of specialist knowledge and skills.

Employers need to ensure that the principles of organisational governance are met to ensure that protected learning, time for reflection and work-based learning and continual professional development opportunities are made available. These features are essential for confidence building and competence development.

Case finding and case management

Case finding refers to a targeted screening method that uses a questionnaire or selected criteria to identify vulnerable people who may be at risk of functional decline but are not in regular contact with either the health or social services. This preventative strategy aims to differentiate individuals on the basis of their problems and to help identify appropriate treatment options in an attempt to assist both planning and demand management services. With regard to medication management, this process will reflect the use of the four trigger questions that can be used as a tool to identify patients who may be socially isolated (see Chapter 4) or physically vulnerable and who may suffer from iatrogenic disease as a result of the adverse effects of prescribed medicines.

Case management can be viewed as 'a proactive, community-based approach to optimise care for older people and ensure the provision of co-ordinated care' (Oboh, 2006, p. 207). This process also aims to target high users of health and social care services with a view to streamlining the care that is offered. This is the remit of the case manager who may be either a case manager or a community matron (DoH, 2005, 2005a). The case manager, who may be a pharmacist or a nurse, should be able to co-ordinate the provision of services offered with respect to medicines management and to help community matrons manage the care of patients, but can also navigate both the health and social care systems to ensure that patients receive the necessary care to successfully manage their condition(s).

For many older people the difficulties of managing complex medication regimens in addition to managing their physical needs can be problematic. The community nurse's role in the care of older people is well established. Much of the care provided centres on the medication management of older people, particularly those that are cognitively impaired and cannot manage their medication regimen. Griffiths et al. (2004) found that community-based nurses were useful in recognising older people who may be at risk of medication mismanagement. These older people were identified and referred to either their GP or pharmacist for medication review. Identifying older people at risk of potential medication mismanagement can help to reduce the quantity of unplanned hospital admissions in the older person age group.

Caseload management is a nurse intervention that has been successfully implemented in the USA. Unutzer et al. (2001) reported on the use of depression nurse specialists to manage the care of patients with depression, using a quality improvement programme. Depression nurse specialists worked in collaboration with medical practitioners to monitor and follow up patients' care, specifically promoting effective medication management and concordance with antidepressant medication. This nurse-led intervention was successful in providing a quality service for patients.

The role of the community matron mirrors that of the depression nurse specialists with respect to the monitoring of patients with long-term conditions and reporting changes in their management to other members of the community team. During case management, the community matron will develop a set of activities to be performed that focus on the comprehensive assessment of the physical, psychological and nursing needs of the individual patient. This process will enable the community matron to detect deterioration in the patient's condition and respond accordingly. Due to the complex nature and longevity of the conditions being treated, it is likely that the community matron will continue to provide the care for the same caseload of patients for the rest of their life.

This mode of working should improve the quality of care provided to older people, as the community matron will act as the key communicator between the patient and the primary care team and social services. This connection can ensure the provision of accurate information about the patient's drug regimen and treatment plan, but can also educate the patient to ensure that they fully understand the treatment that has been prescribed for them, in particular changes to their medication regimen.

Through effective case management, the community matron should be able to:

- assist the prevention of unnecessary admission to hospital
- reduce the duration of stay of hospital inpatients
- improve outcomes for patients
- integrate all elements of care
- improve the quality of life of patients and their ability to function independently
- assist patients and their families to plan future care
- increase patient choice
- improve the terminal care that is offered to patients
- teach patients, carers and their families about the patient's condition(s) and warning signals if the patient is deteriorating, and how to administer, and the timing of, the patient's drugs; and empower patients to take more control over the management of their condition (DoH, 2006a)
- provide continual care rather than an episodic service (DOH, 2006a)
- support people to focus on self care and self management (DOH, 2006a)
- provide proactive, seamless care that is tailor made to meet the needs of the individual patient (DoH, 2006a)
- empower patients to take more control over the management of their condition
- through continuous treatment, monitor patients for potential deterioration in their condition.

Interprofessional working

A central function of the community matron's role is to engage with hospital staff, in particular consultants, discharge planners and ward-based nurses, regarding the discharge arrangements for inpatients being treated for long-term conditions. This will involve recognition of any changes to medication regimens, including the discontinuation or addition of medicines to an existing regimen and future plans that are pertinent to the medication management of patients under their care (Figure 8.2).

Community matrons must work collaboratively with GPs and other members of the primary care team to achieve the best outcomes for patients. The deployment of community matrons will depend on the quantity of high intensity service users and the size of the practice populations. Smaller practices may 'cluster' their resources in a similar manner to community nursing teams.

It is essential that to support the continual development of the community matron's role, PCTs consider how 'they adapt systems and gain

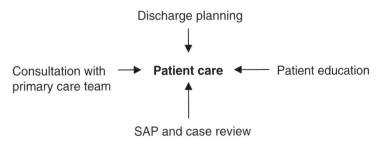

Figure 8.2 Role of the community matron in the medication management of patients with long-term conditions.

commitment from sectors to ensure that the community matron can make referrals, order investigation, admit and discharge patients and secure services such as therapists, social and intermediate care, out of hours teams and have access to patient information' (DoH, 2005, p. 24).

Lay carer's role

One of the key goals of Your Health, Your Care, Your Say (DoH, 2006a) is to increase patient participation in the Expert Patients Programme. The aim of this programme is to educate patients about their chronic disease and to help them develop skills in how to self-care. In addition, a new programme of information giving will be developed that targets patients and their carers and provides an 'information prescription' about the long-term condition, its management, and where they can receive additional peer and self-care support through the available networks.

There are an estimated 6 million carers looking after older people in the UK (DoH, 2006a). Carers are often the main supportive network for vulnerable older people who live alone and have no distant relatives. In this respect, the carer may be the key patient advocate, the orchestrator of care for the patient, and the key communicator who relates the care needed by the patient to other members of the primary care team.

The importance of the medication aspects of long-term conditions is relevant to the carer as well as the patient and their family (Boyle & Chambers, 2000; DoH, 2001b). In many cases, the carer will be responsible for administering the daily concoction of drugs to the patient and therefore needs to be included in all teaching sessions that are given to patients (Banning, 2004). Teaching carers and their patients needs to be structured, informative and based at an appropriate level so that both the carer and the patient understand the importance of administering drugs at the correct time and on a daily basis. In this way the carer can assist the patient's concordance with medication (Banning, 2004a).

Carers are often also the orchestrator of the patient's care and need to be taught how to recognise any side effects arising from specific medicines and why it is important to record this and inform the community matron or another member of the primary care team if these arise. In this way the carer can play an important role in the long-term management of the patient, can encourage adherence to drug regimes and can assist the prevention of unplanned admission to hospital.

The future management of older people with long-term conditions

Currently the care of older people with long-term conditions is managed using a combination of approaches involving community matrons, GP and nurse-led specialist disease operated clinics managed by qualified nurse practitioners, and practice and district nurses who have a non-medical prescribing qualification. This practice is supported by the services offered by the community pharmacist.

The education and training to develop skills in the medication management of patients with long-term conditions focuses on nurses attending specific courses in order to gain either a non-medical prescribing or a community matron qualification. The content of these courses overlaps as they both focus on teaching applied pharmacology and therapeutics, pathophysiology of chronic diseases, the principles of medication management, professional practice and leadership and physical examination of the patient. Although both courses are preparing nurses for complex and extended roles, one significant difference is the academic level; many community matrons already graduates and study for a Master's level community matron qualification, whereas the non-medical prescribing qualification is taught to degree level. In order to prescribe medication, either as an independent or supplementary prescriber, the community matron has to study for a prescribing qualification at a lower academic level than the community matron programme. As prescribing is one of the key professional competences that community matrons have to fulfil, surely this component should have been included in their initial education and training programme.

Nurses who possess an independent prescribing qualification need to study for only two additional days on a non-medical prescribing programme to gain a non-medical prescribing qualification, irrespective of the duration of time since qualifying as an independent nurse prescriber. There are 6,600 independent nurse prescribers in England. Evidence from the evaluation of independent nurse prescribing identified that 14% of the nurse sample of 246 nurses felt inadequately prepared in applied pharmacology and therapeutics and physical examination skills, with a significant minority expressing concerns over their diagnostic ability (DoH, 2005). Similar evidence was generated from an evaluation of the non-medical prescribing course. Hemingway and Davies (2005) reported that mental health nurses with a non-medical prescribing qualification felt that the education and training in psychopharmacology was inadequate. At the time of writing, the non-medical prescribing course is under evaluation. What will the DoH do if the findings that emerge are equivalent to those of the independent nurse prescribing evaluation?

Medical practitioners were alarmed and critical of the addition of opioids to the non-medical prescribing formulary, due to the lack of education and training in disease-specific diagnostics of palliative care nurse prescribers (Mula, 2006). Criticisms such as these could be avoided if nurses were appropriately educated and trained as non-medical prescribers. Firstly, nurses need to be theoretically competent in applied pathophysiology specific to their organ-based speciality. Second, nurses studying for a non-medical prescribing qualification need to undertake a Master's level preparation programme of study that has a strong theoretical and practical focus on physical assessment, clinical diagnostics and clinical reasoning (Banning, 1999), similar to the course provided for community matron education and training.

Surely it is time for the DoH to work with the NMC to reconsider the issue of advanced professional practice in relation to nurse prescribing education (Figure 8.3). There is a need to develop a more progressive programme of education and training in medication management, that meets the learning needs of nurses and encourages nurses with the appropriate scientific foundation to continue their further education at Master's level. This level of knowledge and skills in differential diagnosis, physical assessment and pharmacological

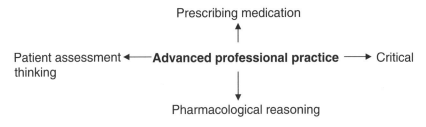

Figure 8.3 Tenets of advanced professional practice.

reasoning will allow nurses to prescribe medication from the BNF (Banning, 1999).

There is a need to include a generic prescribing qualification within the community matron's education and training programme. Community matrons as advanced nurse practitioners will be accredited with a Master's degree in medication management and a recognised prescribing and patient assessment NMC qualification with a five-year renewal agreement. This will ensure the creditability of the qualification, enhance patient safety, and provide some assurance to the public and medical practitioners that community matrons with non-medical prescribing qualifications have the ability and credentials to assess, diagnose and prescribe efficiently and with optimum safety for the patient. This qualification will allow community matrons as non-medical prescribers to seek appropriate financial remuneration for their services.

In terms of the management of long-term conditions, GPs can use practice-based commissioning to employ appropriately qualified non-medical prescribers to manage organ-based speciality clinics at a fraction of the costs of employing a GP. A contractual agreement between the GP and the non-medical prescriber would ensure job security and creditability. Alternatively, the GP could employ a nurse entrepreneur to manage personal medical services. In the UK, the concept of the nurse entrepreneur is steadily evolving as nurses, usually with a community background, offer their services to GPs or Primary Care Trusts as part of the provision of primary care medical services. Some nurse entrepreneurs purchased a general practice and employed a GP to manage patients with complex cases. This consensual arrangement permitted the nurse entrepreneurs to offer personal medical services to patients at flexible times, for example weekends and longer evening surgeries, as identified by the DoH (2006a).

Conclusion

The medication management of long-term medical conditions is a complex and resource intensive activity that is financially draining to NHS budgets. An exacerbation of a long-term condition such as asthma or chronic obstructive airways disease can lead to unplanned admission to hospital, therapeutic intervention, prolonged stay in hospital and continuous follow-up. Measures to control the medication management of long-term conditions, particularly for older people, have been implemented via the Single Assessment Process, non-medical prescribing initiatives, the development and implementation of the community matron role (DoH, 2004c, 2005a) and the Medicines Partnership (2002). These initiatives are still in their infancy and yet could be useful, cost-effective measures that aim to provide an improved service for older people and reduce the financial burden on cash-strapped NHS resources.

Implications for practice

- In the short term, it is the government's intention to train 3,000 community matrons in England to take on patient management roles and to prescribe medication as either a non-medical or independent nurse prescriber. This is in response to the financial demands that older people with long-term conditions exert on the cash-strapped NHS budgets, in particular the cost of prescriptions and medical care. The education and training programme was developed from pilot sites (DoH, 2006). It is unknown whether this programme meets the needs of senior nurses who are either in training or employed as community matrons, as it does not allow nurses to prescribe medication. In order to prescribe, nurses need to study for an additional qualification as a non-medical or independent nurse prescriber. This has proved problematic for some community matrons.
- Long-term implications relate to the need for a more progressive educational structure that will allow nurses to study for a generic prescribing qualification. This would involve the merger of non-medical and independent nurse prescribing programmes with the community matron education and training programme. This Master's-based programme would provide senior nurses with the appropriate scientific background, such as the nurse practitioner, with opportunities to be educated to assess patients, provide a differential diagnosis, prescribe medication and follow up the patient attending an organ-based speciality clinic. This form of training would be recognised by the NMC and would incorporate a five-year assessment structure to ensure the credibility of the qualification for both patients and medical professionals. Nurses working as advanced practitioners could take on entrepreneurial roles that could be beneficial for the future of the NHS and the provision of patient care.
- This educational arrangement would reduce the confusion that exists over the legalities of prescribing practices and the professional accountability associated with nurse prescribing. It would also provide the development of a professional tiered system where levels of accountability were justified and identified, as well as providing a career pathway for community-based nurses.

The community pharmacist's role in the management of older people and their medicines

Jon Waterfield

Learning objectives

After completing this chapter, the reader should be able to:

- outline the new contractual framework for community pharmacists in England and how this may potentially contribute to the management of medicines for older people
- describe some of the opportunities for community pharmacists to become involved in the implementation of the National Service Framework for Older People
- compare and contrast a medicines use review with a medication review
- discuss the role of the community pharmacist in offering a medication management service to care homes for older people
- describe the role of the community pharmacist within a multidisciplinary health care team.

Introduction

The introduction of a new contractual framework for community pharmacists in April 2005 has opened up new opportunities and formalised many established community pharmacy services. There are many opportunities for community pharmacists created by the new contract that will link with the National Service Framework for Older People

(DoH, 2001). A visit to their local pharmacy is an essential weekly routine for many older people. This visit often involves interaction with the pharmacist and their support staff (Figure 9.1).

It is well established that community pharmacists build up strong relationships with older people and their carers when they collect their repeat medication. This regular contact offers the opportunity for the pharmacist to enquire about their medication and general health and discuss any problems that may have arisen since their last visit. The pharmacist also has an active role to play in the informal monitoring of treatment and alerting the patient and prescriber when pharmaceutical intervention becomes necessary.

A large proportion of repeat prescribing and dispensing is for older people. The positive role that a community pharmacist can play in this area has been recognised in the new Community Pharmacy Contractual Framework (DoH, 2004d). The management and dispensing of repeatable NHS prescriptions is an essential service within the new contract. Repeat dispensing offers an alternative way for patients with long-term conditions to obtain repeat supplies of their medicines at their local pharmacy without the need to contact their medical practice every time a new prescription is needed.

The National Service Framework for Older People aims to ensure that older people gain maximum benefit from their medication and also do not suffer unnecessarily from illness caused by excessive,

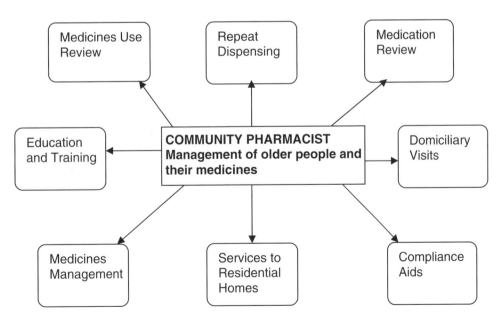

Figure 9.1 The role of the community pharmacist in the management of older people and their medicines.

inappropriate or inadequate consumption of medicines. Community pharmacists may contribute towards this aim by offering an individual medicine use review (MUR). This service is especially suitable for older patients who have long-term conditions such as diabetes, coronary heart disease and asthma. The aim of the MUR is to evaluate how the patient is getting on with their medicines and discuss with the patient if any changes are needed.

Each PCT is authorised to arrange for the provision of additional pharmaceutical services such as services to care homes, medication review services and medicines assessment and compliance support service. These enhanced services are locally commissioned within the new contractual framework. A full level 3 clinical medication review service offers a higher level of pharmaceutical input, and enables the community pharmacist to conduct a review with reference to full patient information. The medication review involves the patient in the decision-making process and makes appropriate referral to other health care professionals.

The National Service Framework for Older People highlights many roles for pharmacists in its implementation. As part of an interprofessional team, the pharmacist has a pivotal role in ensuring that older people gain maximum benefit from their medication. The aim of this chapter is to discuss some key areas of involvement for the community pharmacist in the management of older people and their medicines.

Education and training

The initial training of a pharmacist is a four-year Master of Pharmacy degree course, followed by one year pre-registration training in practice. The pre-registration training is assessed by both competency-based practice assessment and written examination. After registration with the Royal Pharmaceutical Society of Great Britain, the pharmacist is able to practice in either a community or hospital pharmacy. The degree course covers the detailed study of a wide range of subjects including pharmaceutical chemistry, pharmacology, pharmaceutics and pharmacy practice. There is an emphasis on developing clinical skills to equip the pharmacist to contribute fully to patient care within a multidisciplinary team.

On qualification, a wide range of postgraduate development opportunities are available for pharmacists to enhance their clinical and prescribing skills. A pharmacist who aims to work as a supplementary prescriber is required to undertake further training. The government recently announced measures to allow qualified extended formulary nurse prescribers and pharmacist independent prescribers to prescribe any licensed medicine for any medical condition, with the exception of controlled drugs. This means that pharmacists undergoing further training will be able to prescribe independently for the local community. This extension of prescribing responsibility will improve choice and access for patients, and enable more flexible team working within the NHS.

With their specialist knowledge of medicines, pharmacists have a unique role in the training of others involved in patient care. Examples of pharmacist-led training programmes include:

- formulary development and prescribing advice for GPs
- prescribing courses for nurse prescribers
- bespoke medication training courses for carers in the community and residential care homes.

On an individual patient basis, the community pharmacist aims to ensure that the patient is fully informed about their medication. Education and training activities are vital to this patient-centred role.

Community pharmacy contractual framework

For many years pharmacists have been offering a wide range of services directly to the public. The NHS has recognised the important role of pharmacists in delivering pharmaceutical services to the public by introducing a new contractual framework (DoH, 2004d) referred to earlier in this chapter.

There are three tiers of nationally agreed services:

- essential services
- advanced services
- enhanced services.

Essential services are services offered by all community pharmacists. In addition to dispensing NHS prescriptions, the pharmacist will offer the following essential services:

- repeat dispensing
- public health advice
- signposting
- self care
- medicines disposal.

Repeat dispensing will provide more support in the community for people with long-term conditions. GPs will be able to issue a prescription lasting up to a year and the pharmacist will dispense the medication at a convenient time, without the need for a return visit to the GP. The availability of this service will lead to improved patient choice, convenience and the opportunity for an increased level of pharmaceutical care.

The aim of providing public health advice as an essential service is to reduce health inequalities and improve health. For example, the community pharmacist will offer advice on smoking cessation, blood pressure reduction, weight management and nutrition. Through participation in local and national health promotion campaigns, pharmacists will help to tackle national priorities such as obesity, coronary heart disease and cancer. The community pharmacist will be able to offer a signposting service that will help to identify other health service providers and advise the public on where to get appropriate advice. The aim of the self care component of the essential service is to enable people to improve their own health and care for themselves. This is achieved mainly through advice on how to maintain and improve health. Examples include the provision of advice on over-the-counter medicines and associated health care advice. The safe disposal of unwanted medicines is essential to reduce harm to the public and to the environment. The community pharmacist can offer advice and practical options for disposal of unwanted medicines.

The second tier of services within the contractual framework, advanced services, may be provided by pharmacists if both the pharmacist and their premises are accredited. The MUR service already referred to is an example of an advanced service and will be discussed in more detail later in this chapter.

Enhanced services make up the third tier of the national contract. These services are commissioned locally by PCTs to meet community health needs. Pharmacists are commissioned locally to provide services such as smoking cessation, minor ailments schemes and clinics for long-term conditions such as diabetes.

This new contract should enable people to access more health services from their local pharmacist. Of particular relevance to the older person is the availability of repeat dispensing, the MUR service and locally developed enhanced services such as medication reviews. These three services will now be discussed further.

Summary: Potential advantages of the new contract for older people

- Improved patient choice, convenience and access to medicines
- Reduced demand on GPs and other primary care staff – repeat dispensing
- Support for delivery of the GP contract
- Care for people with long-term conditions
- Reduction in health inequalities
- Improved patient safety

Repeat dispensing

It is estimated that repeat prescriptions account for about 75% of all items on a prescription and 81% of prescribing costs in general practice (Harris & Dajada, 1996). The current system of generating repeat prescriptions is time consuming for GPs and their staff and often results in inconvenience for the patient.

For many older people the monthly ritual of ordering their repeat medication can be an onerous task, particularly if the patient is confused and without adequate support. Typically the management of a repeat prescription involves the following stages:

- the patient contacts their GP practice either by telephone or completes a repeat prescription request form marked with the required prescription items
- the GP practice on receiving the request generates a repeat prescription. This process involves the GP signing a new prescription form and in most cases can take up to 48 hours
- the patient collects the repeat prescription from the GP practice
- the prescription is taken to the pharmacy for dispensing.

Many pharmacies offer a prescription collection and delivery service, which helps to simplify this process. In repeat prescription collection services, the patient authorises a named pharmacy to collect their repeat prescription from their GP practice on their behalf. The patient can choose to collect the completed prescription from the pharmacy or opt to have the medication delivered directly to their home. This process is undoubtedly more convenient for the patient as it bypasses some of the stages outlined above. However, one of the disadvantages of home delivery is that there is no direct interaction with the pharmacist to answer patient queries about their repeat medication. With this system the patient still has to remember to order their repeat prescription and must allow sufficient time for the rest of this process. Inevitably problems can arise due to delays in ordering the repeat item or delays in signing the repeat prescription. Typical scenarios with the elderly confused patient include the continuous supply of medication being interrupted, or the patient ordering items that are no longer needed. One of the weaknesses of this system is a lack of compliance checks and inadequate provision of medication reviews.

The new repeat dispensing arrangements offer an alternative way for patients with long-term conditions to obtain repeat supplies of their medication at their local pharmacy, without the need to contact their GP practice every time a new prescription is needed.

Repeat prescriptions have been limited by NHS regulations and reimbursement processes. In April 2004 legislation came into force to enable prescribing doctors, independent nurse prescribers and all supplementary prescribers to issue repeatable prescriptions, and allow pharmacists to dispense and be reimbursed for repeatable prescriptions under the NHS.

For this repeat dispensing system to work, it is important that the patient is selected carefully as this arrangement is not suitable for all patients. Repeat dispensing is more suitable for patients with long-term conditions that are considered likely to remain stable for the duration of the repeat dispensing period. The decision to enter a patient into this system is a joint one between prescriber and the patient. The pharmacist could also input into the decision process based on their knowledge of the patient and the patient's history of managing their repeat medication. If the elderly patient is confused and has numerous medication changes, then they are not a good candidate for repeat dispensing arrangements. However, if the older person has a stable medical condition and has not recently been hospitalised, they may benefit from the new repeat dispensing arrangements. The patient needs to give fully informed consent before participating in the repeat dispensing service, as there is exchange of information about medication and treatment between the prescriber and the pharmacist.

The repeat dispensing prescription consists of a computer-generated repeatable prescription signed by the prescriber and a number of 'batch issues' to enable the pharmacist to dispense the medication in instalments. The batch issue forms are not signed by the prescriber and are used by the pharmacist to supply the medication. This allows a certain amount of flexibility about when the repeat prescription is requested and supplied.

A positive benefit of the new repeat dispensing system is that the pharmacist is fully involved with checking the suitability of the ongoing medication. This is in contrast to the arrangements where repeat prescriptions are issued routinely by administrative staff at the medical practice. Under the new arrangements, before dispensing each instalment of a repeat prescription, pharmacists are required to:

- make sure that the patient is taking the medicines appropriately
- enquire if the patient is suffering from any side effects from their treatment and if necessary refer the patient for a review of their treatment
- check that the patient's medication or health has not changed since the repeatable prescription was issued
- inform the prescriber of any clinically significant issues arising during the period of repeat dispensing.

Summary: Opportunities from repeat dispensing arrangements for the pharmacist to contribute to medicines management issues with the older patient:

- identification of any medicines not being requested
- discuss the overuse of medicines – for example overordering of medicines used on a 'when required' basis
- discuss the underuse of medicines – for example non-compliance with anti-hypertensive medication
- identification of any side effects and related compliance issues
- discuss with the patient the use of each medicine
- check drug therapy monitoring – for example ensuring that the patient is attending for blood pressure monitoring or having the necessary routine tests
- use the opportunity to offer additional advice about specific conditions – for example, osteoporosis and associated health care advice

Medicine use reviews (MURs)

The main aim of the MUR is to improve the patient's knowledge, concordance and use of medicines. This involves establishing the patient's actual use, understanding and experience of taking their medicines. As part of the MUR process, the ineffective use of medicines will be identified and also any side effects that may impact on patient compliance. The MUR service specification (PSNC, 2007) outlines the conditions for this advanced service.

The consultation is normally carried out face to face with the patient in a community pharmacy in a designated consultation area. If for a practical reason a pharmacist wishes to carry out an MUR service in a patient's home or at a day centre, they would need to seek prior approval from the local primary care organisation. An MUR should be conducted with patients on multiple medicines and those with long-term conditions, every 12 months. The patient must have been using the pharmacy for the dispensing of prescriptions for at least the previous three months. The pharmacist can accept referrals for an MUR from other health care professionals or a patient can make an individual request for an MUR. In some situations, the local primary care organisation may identify specific patient groups that would be appropriate for referral for an MUR.

In some cases the requirement for an MUR to be undertaken may be evident from the identification of a significant problem during the dispensing process. This is termed 'prescription intervention' and would be over and above the basic safety interventions which a pharmacist would be involved in as part of the essential dispensing service.

All recommendations from an MUR are made using a nationally agreed reporting template and are communicated to the patient's GP. The MUR report consists of a significant amount of information gathering to determine how the patient is taking their medication. Table 9.1 highlights some examples of common interventions when conducting an MUR with an older patient.

Medication review

One of the main limitations of an MUR is that there is no access to patient notes and the pharmacist is dependent on information provided by the patient and pharmacy medication records. By contrast, a systematic level 3 clinical medication review requires full access to patient notes and prescription history. The majority of evidence for pharmacist-conducted medication reviews, with access to patients and their clinical record, shows a benefit to patients and their clinical

Table 9.1 Typical pharmacist interventions for a medicines use review with an older patient.

Notes from MUR documentation	Pharmacist action point(s)
The patient is only taking their bendroflumethiazide tablets occasionally	Compliance issue – discuss purpose of medication, blood pressure monitoring and reasons for non compliance. Explore use of compliance aid
Analgesics intended to be taken on a when required basis are being taken continuously	Discuss intended doses using patient medication record (PMR) data. Look at suitability of analgesics prescribed for pain and discuss with GP
Multiple paracetamol preparations being prescribed	Ensure patient is aware of maximum dosage of paracetamol and refer to GP to simplify regimen
The patient is unsure or unable to their inhaler use	Demonstrate the correct use of inhaler and spacer devices. Possibility of using a breath actuated device. Refer to asthma clinic for ongoing support
There are problems with the ordering, obtaining and using of medicines	Discuss options available such as repeat prescription collection and delivery services. Determine if the patient is suitable for the repeat dispensing service
Temazepam 10 mg tablets, prescribed one at night when required (quantity 56) – being used regularly every night	Discuss problems associated with regular usage, including risk of falls. Refer to GP to reduce quantity and determine if this medication is still needed
Taking lactulose 5 ml when required, has recently purchased senna tablets and experiencing abdominal cramps	Check medication profile to ensure problem is not drug induced. Counsel on the need for increased fluid intake and discuss lifestyle measures to reduce constipation

record (Petty et al., 2005). The medication review is an enhanced service that is commissioned on a local basis by the primary care organisation.

One specific target within the NSF is a medication review for all patients aged over 75.

All patients in this age group should have their medication reviewed at least annually, and those receiving four or more medicines should be reviewed every six months.

A number of research projects have looked at different formats of medication review (Mackie et al., 1999; Morgan et al., 2000; Krska et al., 2001). Studies have contrasted pharmacists working in a medical practice with full access to patient records, with pharmacists working from pharmacy patient medication record data. When the pharmacist works actively in the medical practice, recommendations were implemented in 50–96% of cases. However, if the feedback from the medication review was of a passive written nature, the implementation rate was much lower at about 20%. An effective way of improving repeat prescribing is to establish a medication review clinic within a medical practice. Patients are selected and an appointment is made to discuss their medication in depth. Another approach is the 'brown bag review' where the patient is asked to bring all the medicines they have at home into the pharmacy. This provides the opportunity to clarify what the patient is taking, what is no longer being taken and a detailed discussion about their medication. This type of review does not use data taken from surgery or pharmacy records.

A medication review for older people receiving more than four medicines is particularly important as it is well established that polypharmacy leads to increased side effects and adverse drug reactions. A full review should also be targeted at patients who have suffered adverse changes in health. For example, if an elderly person has experienced dizzy spells, falls or confusion, it is important to establish if their medication has contributed to the problem. Older patients discharged from hospital are also good candidates for medication review as post-discharge medication problems can arise. For example, a patient or their GP may unintentionally restart medication that has been stopped while in hospital. Another problem may be that there are medication duplication issues, caused by both hospital prescriber and GP. Patients in a residential setting can benefit from a detailed medication review and this is explored in the next section.

A medication review conducted by a community pharmacist is a specific commissioned service and the service specification will determine how patients are selected. The local scheme may target patients based on the number of medicines they are taking, or may include patients within a certain therapeutic area or condition, for example, areas relevant to NSF targets such as patients who have had a fall or are recovering from a stroke.

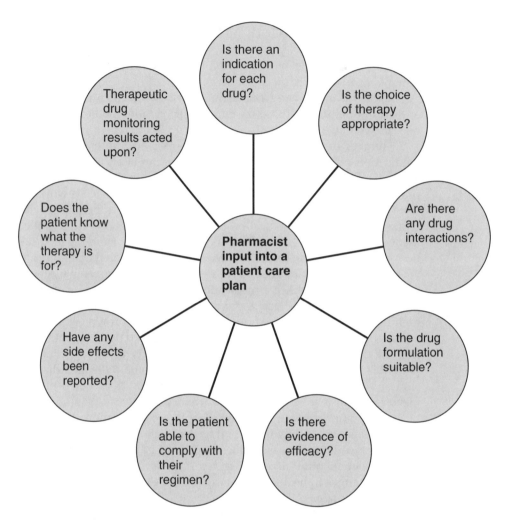

Figure 9.2 Pharmaceutical input into a medication review and the resulting care plan.

From the medication review an individual care plan should be developed. Figure 9.2 outlines some of the pharmaceutical issues that can be considered in the development of the patient care plan.

The availability of a locally driven medication review service with specific entry criteria for older people is another important way that the community pharmacist can contribute to the care of the older population.

Services to residential homes

Community pharmacists offering a medication management service to care homes need to be accredited by their local primary care organisation. An accredited pharmacist can offer a full medication management service to the home, which is documented in a written contract between the home, pharmacist and primary care organisation. Care homes for the older person usually include care of the frail older person or the elderly mentally ill. Pharmacists engaged in providing a pharmaceutical advisory and support service to care homes for older people have a responsibility to ensure that service users receive the same level of support as those who live at home, in terms of meeting the NSF targets for older people.

There are a number of pharmaceutical care issues that are particularly relevant for the frail older person. These issues are a result of the increased use of medicines, together with the age-related pharmacodynamic and pharmacokinetic changes that occur in the elderly. Table 9.2 outlines some of the medication issues for older people in residential care homes.

For the elderly mentally ill, the common mental health conditions include depression, dementias, Alzheimer's disease and anxiety. Pharmaceutical care issues are similar to those seen in the elderly frail person and there is the need for regular medication reviews, especially to check the appropriateness of dosages. It is often difficult to distinguish between the confusion of old age and drug related illness; pharmacists need to be aware of this.

Every residential and care home is required by the National Care Standards Commission to have a written medicines handling policy, and as part of the advisory visit the pharmacist will check that this policy is implemented. The Royal Pharmaceutical Society of Great Britain has prepared guidelines on the use of medicines in residential homes (RPSGB, 2001). This document emphasises the importance of interprofessional working between doctors, community pharmacists

Table 9.2 Some examples of specific medication problems of older people in residential care homes.

Problem	Drug example
Dizziness, drowsiness and confusion	Benzodiazepines and hypnotics have a greater 'hangover effect' Laxatives may be overused and lead to dehydration Diuretics may be used at too high a dose, causing electrolyte imbalance and hypotension Prochloperazine may be prescribed for dizziness without investigating the underlying cause
Incontinence	Aggravated by diuretic medication, appropriate dosage and timing will need to be considered
Renal impairment	Drug choices and dosages need to be adjusted accordingly

and nurses to ensure that the service user obtains maximum benefit from their medicines.

As part of the advisory visit to the care home, the pharmacist should examine the medication profile of individual service users, which includes a detailed record of all medicines taken by the resident.

The medicines handling policy should also cover such areas as self-medication and the use of home remedies. Within a risk management framework, residents who are assessed as able to self-medicate should be encouraged to maintain their independence. The decision regarding self-medication should involve all parties involved with the service user. It is important to involve a pharmacist in the process so that they can contribute to the decision-making process. In many cases of self-medication in the elderly, there are important pharmaceutical issues that can be raised by the pharmacist. For example, assessing the individual medicines for toxicity in overdose, or offering alternative dosage forms that may be more suitable.

The pharmacist visiting the care home will be involved in three main areas:

- any practical issues arising from the medicines policy document, for example problems relating to storage of medicines and record keeping
- any clinical issues relating to individual service users' medication
- any training needs of the care home staff.

A record of the pharmacist visit is provided for the care home manager and the primary care organisation, and any concerns are highlighted. This provides the home with the opportunity to rectify any problems before an official inspection. The pharmacist is required to maintain accurate records of all visits undertaken, and records of all advice given should be available on request.

Monitored dosage systems (MDSs) are useful for patients taking multiple medicines. They were originally designed to improve the administration of medication to the service user by the carer. In a residential home situation, a monitored dosage system offers a convenient and systematic way of managing medicine administration.

The two main types of MDS are:

- Heat-sealed blister packs on a backing card, clearly marked with the day and time of administration. A separate pack is used for each medication and each is stored on a metal rack. The metal racks correspond to different times of administration, for example morning, lunchtime, afternoon and evening.
- Plastic Dosette boxes with separate compartments corresponding to different days and times of administration. Each compartment is enclosed by a plastic seal and contains all the medication to be administered at that time.

For many homes the MDS system is seen as an important aid for managing medicine administration. For the community pharmacist visiting the home and offering advisory support, the system offers a convenient way of assessing compliance with the prescribed medicine and also compliance with medicine administration recording procedures. For example, there may be a pattern of evening doses being missed and it would be important to check the medicine administration record (MAR) sheet to ensure that a reason for not taking the medicine is recorded. The MAR sheet provides valuable information about each service user in terms of their compliance with their prescribed medicine, and in some cases it is necessary to arrange a full medication review.

Swallowing difficulties

The swallowing of solid dose forms can present a problem to elderly patients. This may become evident during a routine conversation with an elderly client when supplying their repeat medication or it may be in response to a query from a GP, nurse or care worker in a residential home.

The widespread practice of crushing tablets and opening capsules is of particular concern (Wright, 2002). In some cases the crushing of solid dose forms (tablets and capsules) that have an enteric coating or slow release properties may result in overdose or harm to the patient. This issue also has legal implications as crushing a tablet or opening a capsule means that the medicine is being administered outside the terms of the product licence. Under the Medicines Act 1968, only medical and dental practitioners can authorise the use of unlicensed medicines in humans. Administering an unlicensed medicine removes the protection provided by the Consumer Protection Act 1987 and would mean that the person altering the medication would be personally liable for any harm caused.

If there is a swallowing difficulty, the preferred option is to find a suitable liquid dose form, or investigate the possibility of using a different dosage form that is acceptable to the patient. For example, the medication may be available as liquid or granules or in the form of suppositories. The pharmacist can also check the feasibility of providing the medicine as a special extemporaneously dispensed preparation. This option is not always possible due to a lack of pharmaceutical stability or prohibitive cost.

If an alternative formulation is not available and crushing the dose form appears to be the only option, the next stage is to check if the medicine can be safely crushed or opened. For example, it would be inappropriate for hormonal, cytotoxic or steroidal drugs to be crushed as the powder may go into the air and present a risk to the person administering the dose.

If a decision is made to crush a tablet or open a capsule, then permission is required from the prescriber as medication is being administered in an unlicensed form. In addition, it is good practice to obtain written consent from the patient or their representative, and if the patient is in a care home a record should be made in their care plan. The crushing of tablets is seen as a last resort, and a clear written record of the decision is required for future reference.

If the patient has a percutaneous endoscopic gastrostomy (PEG) tube there are other issues to consider, as most medicines are not licensed for administration by this route. The pharmaceutical issues that would need to be considered are:

- Is the liquid dose equivalent to the solid dose?
- Will the tube become blocked and what flushing out procedure should be used?
- Does the liquid contain sorbitol and is this in sufficient quantity to cause diarrhoea?
- Is the medication light or water sensitive?
- Will the medicines interact directly with the enteral feed?

Swallowing difficulties can present a significant problem to all those involved in the care of an elderly patient. The pharmaceutical input from a community pharmacist can be invaluable in such cases.

Domiciliary visiting schemes

Many elderly patients who would benefit from the advice of a community pharmacist are unable to leave their home and visit the pharmacy. A number of pilot domiciliary visiting schemes for pharmacists to visit patients in their own homes have been introduced. Some studies on the impact of domiciliary visits have demonstrated improved compliance, better storage and ordering procedures and fewer GP consultations (Begley et al., 1997; Lowe et al., 2000).

Domiciliary schemes vary in their patient entry criteria and would typically include patients over 75, living alone, housebound and identified by their medical practice as being at risk of poor compliance. The support offered by the pharmacist on a domiciliary visit is similar to a medication review but takes a broader view of the patient's circumstances and factors affecting their medication.

A typical domiciliary scheme involves four stages:

- initial assessment visit
- preparation of a medication review and pharmaceutical care plan – using information obtained from the patient and liaison with the GP

- follow-up visit including the delivery of any compliance aids
- implementation of a care plan by the pharmacist and GP and patient monitoring at regular intervals.

Compliance aids

For some elderly patients living in the community, a monitored dosage system may be useful to reduce medication errors and improve compliance. Some patients develop their own system and transfer tablets into separately labelled containers for each day of the week. A pharmacist undertaking a domiciliary visit is likely to encounter a range of home-made systems designed to help the patient remember to take the tablets at the appropriate time. In some cases, patients transfer their own medicine into their own compliance aid or may rely on a carer or relative to carry out this role.

A more robust system is to obtain a sealed monitored dosage system from the supplying pharmacy. This may take the form of a filled Nomad® Cassette or a sealed blister packed unit containing seven days' medication. For older patients this may be a useful way of improving compliance, especially if used in conjunction with an MAR sheet.

Physical problems

The community pharmacist is also experienced in helping older people to overcome physical barriers that have a negative effect on taking their medication.

Common interventions include the production of large-print medicine labels for the visually impaired and the use of spacer devices for metered dose aerosols, to overcome problems with co-ordination. The use of a non-child resistant container (CRC) can remove the frustrating barrier of opening a medicine container for a frail elderly person. Supply of a CRC is a legal requirement unless the patient or prescriber specifically requests a non-CRC. Foil blister packs may also present a problem and alternative ways of packaging and presenting medicines for older people need to be considered. For the elderly person with arthritis, the use of a lever device to press an aerosol inhaler can be useful as it enables the patient to activate the device with considerably less effort. If the patient has a large volume of liquid medicine, they may be unable to manage heavy glass bottles and may find smaller plastic bottles more manageable. Self-administration of eye drops is especially difficult and the use of an Autodrop device may be useful. All of these simple practical measures can help support the elderly person to manage their medicines more easily on their own.

Prescribing support

The community pharmacist can offer prescribing support and advice to a range of health care professionals. This may be formal employment with a local medical practice where the pharmacist is actively involved in formulary development, prescribing policy and treatment priorities. Alternatively, it may be an informal relationship that the pharmacist builds up with local GPs, nurses and other health care professionals in response to individual prescriptions.

Prescribing support is particularly relevant in working towards the NSF targets relating to stroke, mental health and falls. Figure 9.3 provides an overview of ways in which the prescribing support pharmacist can input into these areas.

The control of hypertension within specified limits and anti-thrombotic treatment in patients with atrial fibrillation are seen as key interventions to prevent stroke. A pharmacist engaged in prescribing support can contribute to this important target. The prescribing of antipsychotics and benzodiazepines needs to be monitored and reviewed according to local policy. The appropriate prescribing of antidepressants for older people is also a key issue (Donaghue et al., 1998). It is important that prescribing support pharmacists work towards ensuring that prescribing for older people is in accordance with the published guidelines. Patients that have had a fall and are taking medicines known to contribute to falls should have a medication review (Swift, 2001; Feder et al., 2000). Polypharmacy in general is known to be a risk factor for falls, and the prescribing of

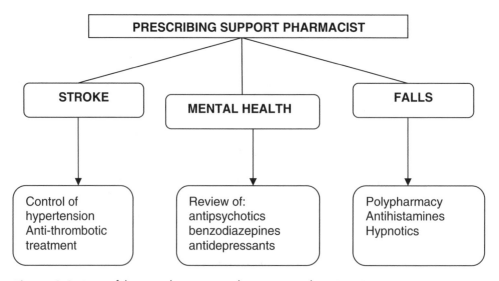

Figure 9.3   Input of the prescribing support pharmacist into the NSF 243 targets.

antihypertensive medication, tricyclic antidepressants, benzodiazepines and antihistamines should be closely monitored. Hypnotics and
tranquillisers are known to contribute to falls in older patients, especially during the night. If an elderly patient is taking diuretics or laxa-
tives, then possible dehydration could be considered to be a risk factor
for falls.

The prescribing support pharmacist within a local medical practice
or primary care organisation is a useful contact for all those concerned
with medication management issues in the elderly.

Multi-disciplinary working

To work efficiently towards the NSF standards and provide improved
services for older people, health care professions will need to develop
strong working partnerships. It is important that pharmacists develop
links with local groups such as NSF implementation groups, clinical
governance frameworks and local Health Improvement Modernisation
Plans.

When an elderly person is discharged from hospital, often with significant changes to their medication, there can be a delay in communication between the hospital and the patient's GP. Some schemes exist
where the hospital pharmacy liaises directly with the patient's nomi-
nated community pharmacy, to ensure they are fully aware of their
discharge medication. This system ensures that when the first post-
discharge prescription is presented, the pharmacist is working with
updated information.

It is important for pharmacists to develop strong links with community-based nurses, local GPs and their support teams. Collaborative
working and shared information help to achieve a more coherent and
comprehensive outcome for the older patient.

Conclusion

The community pharmacist role is multi-faceted and involves providing essential, enhanced and advanced services, undertaking medication review, providing prescribing support to members of the health
care team and multi-disciplinary working with nurses managing
patients in both care and residential homes.

Implications for practice

After reading this chapter it would be useful to consider the following
questions:

Continued

- Would any of my patients benefit from a repeat dispensing service or a medicines use review?
- Do any of my patients have swallowing difficulties and find it difficult to take their prescribed medication?
- Do any of my patients have physical problems or memory difficulties that affect the way that they take their medication?
- How could I work more closely with a community pharmacist in the implementation of the NSF for Older People?

Discuss your answers to the above questions with a community pharmacist.

References

Alibhai, S.M.H. & Naglie, G. (1999) Medication education of acutely hospitalized older patients. *Journal of General Internal Medicine*, **14**, 610–616.

Allan, E.L. & Barker, K.N. (1990) Fundamentals of medication error research. *American Journal of Hospital Pharmacy*, **47** (15), 555–571.

Allard, A., Herbert, R., Rioux, M., Asselin, J. & Voyer, L. (2001) Peer prescription review had no effect on potentially inappropriate prescriptions for the elderly. *Canadian Medical Association Journal*, **164**, 1291–1296.

Andrew, D. & Aspinall, R. (2002) Age-associated thymic atrophy is linked to a decline in IL-7 production. *Experimental Gerontology*, **37** (2), 455–463.

Appelgate, W.B. (2002) Elderly patients' adherence to statin therapy. *JAMA*, **288**, 495–498.

Aronson, J. (1999) Drug excretion: what the prescriber should know. *Prescriber*, October, 67–75.

ASHP (1993) American Society of Health-System Pharmacists Guidelines on Preventing Medication Errors in Hospitals. *American Journal of Hospital Pharmacy*, **50** (12), 305–314.

Asplund, R., Sundberg, B. & Bengtsson, P. (1998) Desmopressin for the treatment of polyuria in the elderly: a dose titration study. *British Journal of Urology*, **82**, 642–646

Atkin, P.A., Finnegan, T.P., Ogle, S.J. & Shenfield, G.M. (1994) Functional ability of patients to manage medication packaging: a survey of geriatric inpatients. *Age and Ageing*, **23**, 113–116.

Attilo, R.M. (1996) Caring enough to understand: the road to oncology medication error prevention. *Hospital Pharmacy*, **31**, 17–26.

Banning, M. (1999) Education, education, education. In: Jones, M. (ed.) *Nurse Prescribing: Politics to Practice*. Balliere Tindall, Oxford.

Banning, M. (2003) Pharmacology education: a theoretical framework of applied pharmacology and therapeutics. *Nurse Education Today*, **23**, 459–466.

Banning, M. (2004) 'An illuminative evaluation of the teaching and learning experience of participant's teaching and studying on an independent nurse prescribing course.' Unpublished EdD thesis. Brunel University, London.

Banning, M. (2004a) Enhancing concordance with prescribed medication in older people. *Nursing Older People*, **16**, 14–17.

Banning, M. (2005) Medication errors: considerations for nurse prescribers. *Nurse Prescribing*, **3** (2), 68–72.

Barat, I., Andreasen, F. & Damsgaard, E.M.S. (2001) Drug therapy in the elderly: what doctors believe and patients actually do. *British Journal of Clinical Pharmacology*, **51**, 615–622.

Barber, N. (2004) Designing information technology to support prescribing decision making. *Quality and Safety in Health Care*, **13** (6), 450–454.

Barber N. & Dean, B. (1998) The incidence of medication errors and ways to reduce them. *Clinical Risk*, **4** (2), 103–106.

Barber, N., Rawlins, M.D. & Dean, F.B. (2003) Reducing prescribing error: competence, control and culture. *Quality and Safety in Health Care*, **12** (suppl 1), 29–32.

Barker, K.N. & McConnell, W.E. (1962) The problems of fetching medication errors in hospitals. *American Journal of Hospital Pharmacy*, **19** (1), 360–369.

Barrett, J. (2005) Rehabilitation bed survey. England council update. *BGS Newsletter online*. March 2005. http://www.bgsnet.org.uk

Bates, D.W. (2001) Reducing medication errors. *JAMA*, **266** (17), 2091–2092.

Bates, D.W., Boyle, D.L., Vander, V.M.B., Schneider, J. & Leape, L.L. (1995) Relationship between medication errors and adverse drug events. *Journal of General Internal Medicine*, **10** (4), 199–205.

Batty, G.M., Grant, R.L., Aggarwal, R., Lowe, D., Potter, J.M., Pearson, M.G. & Jackson, H.D. (2003). Using prescribing indicators to measure the quality of prescribing in elderly medical in-patients. *Age and Ageing*, **32**, 292–298.

Beach, T., Potter, P., Kuo, Y., Emmerling, M.R., Durham, R.A., Webster, S.D., Walker, D.G., Sue, L.I., Scott, S., Layne, K.J. & Roher, A.E. (2000) Cholinergic deafferentation of the rabbit cortex: a new animal model Abeta deposition. *Neuroscience letters*, **283**, 9–12.

Beasley, C. (2005) 'Community matrons will make a difference to patients' lives.' Chief Nursing Officer press release. Department of Health, London.

Beers, M.H. (1992) Medication use in the elderly. In: Calkins, E., Ford, A.B., Katz, P.R. (eds) *Practice of Geriatrics*, 2nd edn, pp. 33–49. W.B. Saunders, Philadelphia.

Beers, M.H. (1997) Explicit criteria for determining inappropriate medication use by the elderly. *Archives of Internal Medicine*, **157**,1531–1536.

Begley, S., Livingstone, C., Hodges, N. & Williamson V. (1997) Impact of domiciliary pharmacy visits on medication management in an elderly population. *International Journal of Pharmacy Practice*, **5**, 111–121.

Bender, A. (1968) Effect of age on intestinal absorption: implications for drug absorption in the elderly. *Journal of the American Geriatrics Society*, **16**, 1331–1339.

Benner, J.S., Glynn, R., Mogun, H., Neumann, P.J., Weins, M.C. & Avorn, J. (2002) Long-term resistance in use of statin therapy in elderly patients. *JAMA*, **288**, 255–262.

Bernett, G.B., Feldman, S., Harlan, M., Smith, B. & Raineri, B.D. (2003) An opportunity for medication risk reduction, healthcare provider collaboration and improved patient care: a retrospective analysis of osteoporosis management. *Journal of American Medical Directors Association*, **4** (6), 329–336.

Bero, L., Lipton, H. & Bird, J. (1991) Characterisation of geriatric drug-related hospital admissions. *Medical Care*, **29**, 989–1003.

Boyle, E. & Chambers, M. (2000) Medication compliance in older individuals with depression: gaining the views of family carers. *Journal of Psychiatric Mental Health Nursing*, **7**, 515–522.

Braak, E. & Braak, H. (1997) Alzheimer's disease: transiently developing dendritic changes in pyramidal cells of sector CA 1 of the Ammon's horn. *Acta Neuropathologica*, **93** (4), 323–325.

Bressler, R. & Bahl, J. (2003) Principles of drug therapy for the elderly patient. *Mayo Clinic Proceedings*, **78**, 1564–1577.

British Geriatrics Society (2004) Intermediate care: guidance for commissioners and providers of health and social care. http://www.bgs.org.uk/publications

Brody, H. (1955) Organization of the cerebral cortex. III. A study of aging in the human cerebral cortex. Journal of Comparative Neurology, **102**, 511–516.

Bruce, J. & Wong, I. (2001) Parenteral medication administration errors by nursing staff on an acute medical admissions ward during day duty. *Drug safety*, **24** (11), 855–862.

Burke, K.M., LeMone, P. & Mohn-Brown, E.L. (2003) *Medical-Surgical Nursing Care*. Prentice Hall, New Jersey.

Burke, S.N. & Barnes, C.A. (2006) Neural plasticity in the ageing brain. *Nature*, **7**, 30–40.

Byetheway, B., Johnson, J., Heller, T. & Muston, R. (2000) 'The management of long-term medication by older people.' Report to the DoH, London.

Cargill, J.M. (1992) Medication compliance in elderly people: influencing variables and interventions. *Journal of Advanced Nursing*, **17**, 422–426.

Carter, S. (2004) Medicines management: opportunities for pharmacists in a new GMS contract. *The Pharmaceutical Journal*, **272** (7291), 350–351.

Castegna, A., Thongboonkerd, V., Klein, J., Lynn, B., Wang, Y. & Osaka, H. et al. (2004) Proteomic analysis of brain proteins in the gracile axonal dystrophy (gad) mouse, a syndrome that emanates from dysfunctional ubiquitin carboxyl-terminal hydrolase L-1, reveals oxidation of key proteins. *Journal of Neurochemistry*, **88** (6), 1540–1546.

Challiner, Y., Carpenter, G.I., Potter, J. & Maxwell, C. (2003) Performance indicators for hospital services for older people. *Age and Ageing*, **32**, 343–346.

Charatan, F. (1999) Family compensated for death after illegible prescription. *BMJ*, **319** (7223), 1456.

Cheek, J. (1997) Nurses and the administration of medications: broadening the focus. *Clinical Nursing Research*, **6**, 253–275.

Chen, J. (1999) Medication concordance is best helped by improving consultation skills. *BMJ*, **318** (7184), 670.

Chin, P. (1986) Medication error prevention. *Nursing*, **16** (12), 36–39.

Clark, W.R. (1999) *A Means to an End: The Biological Basis of Aging and Death*. Oxford University Press, Oxford.

Cline, C.M.J., Björck-Linné, A.K., Israelsson, B.Y.A., Willenheimer, R.B. & Erhardt, L.R. (1999) Non-compliance and knowledge of prescribed medication in elderly patients with heart failure. *European Journal of Heart Failure*, **1** (2), 145–149.

Close, A. (1988) Patient education: a literature review. *Journal of Advanced Nursing*, **13**, 203–213.

Cockcroft, D.W. & Gault, M.H. (1976) Predicator of creatinine clearance from serum creatinine. *Nephron*, **16** (1), 31–41.

Cohen, J.S. (2000) Avoiding adverse drug reactions: effective lower-dose therapies for older patients. *Geriatrics*, **55** (2), 54–64.

Col, N., Fanale, J.E. & Kronholm, P. (1990) The role of medication non-compliance and adverse drug reactions in hospitalisations of the elderly. *Archives of Internal Medicine*, **150**, 841–845.

Cooper, J.W. (1999) Adverse drug reactions-related hospitalisations of nursing care facility patients: a four-year study. *Southern Medical Journal*, **92**, 485–490.

Corkadel, L. & McGlashen, R. (1983) A practical approach to patient teaching. *Journal of Continuing Education in Nursing*, **14**, 9–15.

Cousins, D. & Upton, D. (1994) Medication errors. Watch out for drug name abbreviations. *Pharmacy in Practice*, **4**, 28.

Coyle, J., Price, D., Delong, M. (1983) Alzeimer's disease: a disease of cortical cholinergic innervation. *Science*, **219**, 1184–1190.

Cross, C., Halliwell, E., Borish, W., Pryor, W., Ames, B., Saul, R., McCord, J. & Harman, D. (1987) Oxygen radicals and human disease. *Annals of Internal Medicine*, **107**, 526–545.

Cunningham, G., Dodd, T., Grant, D., McMurdo, M. & Richards, R. (1997) Drug-related problems in elderly patients admitted to Tayside hospitals, methods for prevention and subsequent reassessment. *Age and Ageing*, **26**, 375–382.

Dartnell, J., Anderson, R. & Chohan, V. (1996) Hospitalisation for adverse effects related to drug therapy: incidence, avoidability and costs. *The Medical Journal of Australia*, **164**, 659–662.

Davies, L., Wolska, B. & Hilbich, C. (1988) A4 amyloid protein deposition and the diagnosis of Alzheimer's disease: prevalence in aged brains determined by immunocytochemistry compared with conventional neuropathological techniques. *Neurology*, **38**, 1688–1693.

Davis, S. (1991) Self-administration of medicines. *Nursing Standard*, **5**, 29–31.

Davydov, L., Caliendo, G., Mehl, B. & Smith, L.G. (2004) Investigation of correlation between house-staff work hours and prescribing errors. *American Journal of Health-System Pharmacy*, **61** (11), 1130–1134.

Dean, B., Barber, N. & Schafer, M. (2000) What is a prescribing error? *Quality and Safety in Health Care*, **9**, 232–237.

Dean, B., Schacter, M., Vincent, C. & Barber, N. (2002) Causes of prescribing errors in hospital inpatients: a prospective study. *Lancet*, **359** (9315), 1373–1378.

Dharmarajan, T.S. & Ugalino, J.A. (2001) Understanding the pharmacology of ageing. *Geriatric Medicine Board Review Manual*, **1** (4), 1–12.

Dobrzanski, S., Hammond, I., Khan, G. & Holdsworth, H. (2002) The nature of hospital prescribing errors. *British Journal of Clinical Governance*, **7**, 187–193.

DoH (2000) *The NHS Plan: A plan for investment. A plan for reform.* Department of Health, London.

DoH (2000a) *Raising Standards for Patients: New Partnerships in Out of Hours Care.* Medicines Management Collaborative, London.

DoH (2000b) *An Organisation with a Memory.* Department of Health, London.

DoH (2000–2002) Statistics of prescriptions dispensed in the Family Health Service Authorities: England, 1989–1999. *Statistical Bulletin.* Department of Health, London.

DoH (2001) *National Service Framework for Older People.* Department of Health, London.

DoH (2001a) *National Service Framework for Older People; Medicines and Older People.* Department of Health, London.

DoH (2001b) *Building a Safer NHS for Patients; Implementing An Organisation With a Memory.* Department of Health, London.

DoH (2001c) *Medicines and Older People; Implementing Medicines – Related Aspects of the NSF for Older People.* Department of Health, London.

DoH (2002) *Delivering the NHS Plan; Next Steps On Investment, Next Steps On Reform.* Department of Health, London.

DoH (2002a) Health Service Circular/Local Authority Circular HSC 2002/001; LAC 2002 (1). 'Guidance on the Single Assessment Process for Older People.' Department of Health, London.

DoH (2003) *Care Homes For Older People; National Minimum Care Standards*, 3rd edition. The Stationery Office, London.

DoH (2004) *Building a Safer NHS for patients; Improving Medication Safety.* Department of Health, London.

DoH (2004a) *Management of Medicines – a Resource to Support Implementation of the Wider Aspects of Medicines Management for the National Service Frameworks for Diabetes, Renal services and Long term conditions.* Department of Health, London.

DoH (2004b) *Chronic disease management: A compendium of information.* Department of Health, London.

DoH (2004c) *The NHS Improvement Plan: Putting people at the heart of public services.* Department of Health, London.

DoH (2004d) 'The new contractual framework for community pharmacy.' Department of Health, London.

DoH (2005) 'An NHS and Social care model for improving care for people with long-term conditions.' Department of Health, London.

DoH (2005a) *Supporting People With Long Term Conditions; Liberating the Talents of Nurses Who Care for People With Long Term Conditions.* Department of Health, London.

DoH (2005b) *Supporting People With Long Term Conditions; An NHS & Social Care Model to Support Local Innovation and Integration.* Department of Health, London.

DoH (2005c) 'Nurse and pharmacist prescribing powers extended.' Department of Health, London.

DoH (2005d) *Case Management Competences Framework for the Care of People with Long Term Conditions.* NHS Modernisation Agency and Skills for Health. Department of Health, London.

DoH (2005e) *The Future Direction of the NHS Modernisation Agency (2004).* Department of Health, London.

DoH (2006) 'Nurse prescribers' extended formulary: Additional controlled drugs from January 6th 2006.' http://www.doh.gov.uk/nurse

DoH (2006a). *Our Health, Your Care, Your Say.* Department of Health, London.

DoH (2006b) 'Caring for people with long term conditions: an education framework for community matrons and case managers.' Department of Health, London.

DoH (2006c) 'A new ambition for old age: Next steps in implementing the national service framework for older people.' Department of Health, London.

DoH (2006d) Orders and regulations relating to the use of nationwide rollout of electronic prescribing service. Department of Health, London.

Donaghue, J., Katona, C. & Tylee, A. (1998) The treatment of depression: antidepressant prescribing for elderly patients in primary care. *Pharmaceutical Journal,* **260**, 500–502.

Doraiswamy, P. & Xiong, G. (2006) Pharmacological strategies for the prevention of Alzheimer's disease. *Expert Opinion on Pharmacotherapy,* **7** (1), 1–10.

Douglas, J., Bax, R. & Munro, J. (1980) The pharmacokinetics of cerfuroxime in the elderly. *Journal of Antimicrobial Chemotherapy,* **6**, 543–549.

Duggan, C., Feldman, R., Hough, J. & Bates, I. (1998) Reducing adverse prescribing discrepancies following hospital discharge. *International Journal of Pharmacy Practice,* **6** (2), 77–82. Cited DoH (2004a) *Management of Medicines a Resource To Support Implementation Of The Wider Aspects Of Medicines Management for the National Service Frameworks for Diabetes, Renal services and Long term conditions.* Department of Health, London.

Dummett, S. (1998) Avoiding drug administration errors: The way forward. *Nursing Times,* **94** (30), 58–60.

Ellenbecker, C.H. (2004) Nurses' observations and experiences of problems and adverse effects of medication management in home care. *Geriatric Nursing,* **25**, (3), 164–170.

Eriksson, C.E. (1984). Cardiac drugs in the elderly. In Vestra, R.E. Ed. *Drug Treatment in the Elderly.* Sydney; ADIS Health Science Press.

Esposito, L. (1995) The effects of medication education on adherence to medication regimens in an elderly population. *Journal of Advanced Nursing,* **21**, 935–943.

Evans, M. Triggs, E. & Broe, G. (1980) Systemic availability of orally administered L-dopa in the elderly Parkinsonian patient. *European Journal of Clinical
Pharmacology*, **17**, 215–221.

Faber, J., Azzunguni, M., Di Romana, S. & Vanhaeverbeek, M. (1991) Fatal
confusion between losec and lasix (Letter). *Lancet*, **337**, 1286–1287.

Feder, G., Cryer, C., Donovan, S. & Carter, S. (2000) Guidelines for the prevention of falls in people over 65. *BMJ*, **321**, 1007–1011.

Forbes, G. & Reina, J. (1970) Adult lean mass declines with age: some longitu-
dinal observations. *Metabolism*, **19**, 653–663.

Ford, G.A. (2000) Pharmacodynamics. In: Crome, P. & Ford, G. (eds) *Drugs and
the Older Population*, pp 90–108. Imperial College Press, London.

Foster, T.C. & Norris, C.M. (1997) Age associated changes in Ca^{2+} dependent processes: relation to hippocampal synaptic plasticity. *Hippocampus*, **7**, 602–612.

Franceschi, C., Bonafe, M. & Valensin, S. (2000) Human immunosenescence:
the prevailing of innate immunity, the failing of clonotypic immunity and
the filling of immunological space. *Vaccine*, **18**, 1717–1720.

Furlong, S. (1996) Do programmes of medicine self-administration enhance
patient knowledge, compliance and satisfaction? *Journal of Advanced Nursing*,
23, 1254–1262.

Gardener, E.M. & Murasko, D.M. (2002) Age-related changes in Type 1 and
Type 2 cytokine production in humans. *Biogerontology*, **3** (5), 271–290.

Gilbert, A.L., Roughead, E.E., Beilby, J., Mott, K. & Barratt, J.D. (2002) Collaborative medication management services: improving patient care. *The Medical
Journal of Australia*, **177** (4), 189–192.

Ginaldi, L. & Sternberg, H. (2002) The immune system. In: Timiras, P. (ed.)
Physiological Basis of Aging and Geriatrics, pp. 265–283. CRC Press, Boca
Raton, FL.

Glazer-Waldman, H., Hall, K. & Weiner, M.F. (1985) Patient education in a
public hospital. *Nursing Research*, **34**, 184–185.

Gleason, M.S. (1996) Pharmacologic issues in aging. *Critical Care Nursing Quar-
terly*, **19**, 7–12.

GMSC (1989) *NHS General Medical Services Regulations*, para 34, (2)b. General
Medical Services Committee, London.

Gold, D.R., Rogacz, S. & Bock, N. (1992) Rotating shift work, sleep and acci-
dents related to sleepiness in hospital nurses. *American Journal of Public
Health*, **82** (7), 1011–1014.

Goldbeck-Wood, S. (1996) Medical defence union exposes drug errors. *British
Medical Journal*, **312**, 1439.

Goldstein, R., Hulme, H. & Willits, J. (1998) Reviewing repeat prescribing –
general practitioners and community pharmacists working together. *International Journal of Pharmacy Practice*, **6**, 60–66.

Grant, R.L., Aggarwal, R. & Lowe, D. (2002) National sentinel clinical audit of
evidence-based prescribing for older people: methodology and development. *Journal of Evaluation in Clinical Practice*, **8**, 189–198.

Gray, R., Wykes, T. & Gournay, K. (2003) The effect of medication management
training on community mental health nurse's clinical skills. *International
Journal of Nursing Studies*, **40**, 163–169.

Griffith, S. (1990). A review of the factors associated with patient compliance and the taking of prescribed medicines. *British Journal of General Practice*, **40**, 114–116.

Griffiths, R. (2004) A nursing intervention for the quality use of medicines by elderly community clients. *International Journal of Nursing Studies*, **10** (4), 166–174.

Guardian (1988) Pharmacist: GP blamed for coma. *The Guardian* newspaper, 17 March.

Guzowski, J.F. Lyford, G.L., Stevenson, G.D., Houston, F.P., McGaugh, J.L., Worley, P.F. & Barnes, C.A. (2000) Inhibition of activity-dependent arc protein expression in the rat hippocampus impairs the maintenance of long term potentiation and the consolidation of long term memory. *Journal of Neuroscience*, **20**, 3993–4001.

Hall, K.E. (2003) Effect of aging on gastrointestinal function. In: Hazzard, W.R., Andres, R., Bierman, E.L. & Blass, J.P. (eds) *Principles of Geriatric Medicine and Gerontology*, 5th edn, pp. 593–600. McGraw-Hill, New York.

Hames.A. & Wynne, H.A. (2001) Unlicensed and off-label drug use in elderly people. *Age and Aging*, **30**, 530–531.

Hammerlein, A., Derendorf, H. & Lowenthal, D.T. (1998) Pharmacokinetic and pharmacodynamic changes in the elderly. Clinical implications. *Clinical Pharmacokinetics*, **35**, 49–64.

Harris, C.M. & Dajada, R. (1996) The scale of repeat prescribing. *British Journal of General Practice*, **46**, 649–653.

Hartley, G.M. & DoHillon, S. (1998) An observational study of the prescribing and administration of intravenous drugs in a general hospital. *International Journal of Pharmacy Practice*, **6** (8), 38–45.

Hemingway, S. & Davies, J. (2005) Non-medical prescribing education provision: How do we meet the needs of the diverse nursing specialisms? www.nurse-prescriber.co.uk.

Henderson, J., Goldacre, M.J., Graveney, M.J. & Simmons, H.M. (1989) Use of medical record linkage to study readmission rates. *BMJ*, **299**, 209–213.

Hensley, K., Hall, N., Subramaniam, R., Cole, P., Harris, M., Aksenov, M., et al. (1995) Brain regional correspondence between Alzheimer's disease histopathology and biomarkers of protein oxidation. *Journal of Neurochemistry*, **65** (5), 2146–2156.

Hill, P. & Ball, D. (1992) Self-medication for elderly care. *Care of the Elderly*, October, 405–407.

Hilmer, S.N, Cogger, V.C., Fraser, R., McLean, A.J., Sullivan, D. & Le Couteur, D.G. (2005) Age-related changes in the hepatic sinusoidal endothelium impede lipoprotein transfer in the rat. *Hepatology*, **42** (6), 1349–1354.

Hoffman, J.M. & Proulx, S. (2003) Medication errors caused by confusion of drug names. *Drug Safety*, **28**, 445–452.

Holloway, A. (1996) Patient knowledge and information concerning medication on discharge from hospital. *Journal of Advanced Nursing*, **24**, 1169–1174.

Honer, M. & Lancaster, T. (1996) Who needs antiplatelet therapy? *British Journal of General Practice*, **46**, 367–370.

Hopps, L. (1983) A case for patient teaching. *Nursing Times*, **48**, 42–45.

Hughes, A., Daniel, S., Blankson, S. & Lees, A. (1993) A clinicopathologic study of 100 cases of Parkinson's disease. Archives of Neurology, **50**, 140–148.

Hulka, B.S., Cassel, J.C., Kupper, L.L. & Burdette, J.A. (1976) Communication, compliance, and concordance between physicians and patients with pre-scribed medications. *American Journal of Public Health*, **66**, 847–853.

Husse, B., Sopart, A. & Isenberg, G. (2003) Cyclical stretch-induced apoptosis from young rats but necrosis in myocytes from old rats. *American Journal of Physiology – Heart and Circulatory Physiology*, **285** (4), 1521–1527.

Hutton, M. (2003) Calculations for new prescribers. *Nursing Standard*, **17** (25), 47–55.

Jackson, S.H.D. (1995) Prescribing for elderly patients. *Hospital Update*, September, 388–393.

Jenkins, D. (1993) The quality of written inpatient prescriptions. *International Journal of Pharmacy Practice*, **2** (3), 176–179.

Jones, M.W., Errington, M.L., French, P.J., Fine, A., Bliss, T.V.P., Garel, S., Charnay, P., Bozon, B., Laroche, S. & Davis, S. (2001) A requirement for the immediate early gene *Zif268* in the expression of late LTP and long term memories. *Nature Neuroscience*, **4**, 289–296.

Julien, R. (1995) *A primer of drug action. A concise nontechnical guide to the actions, uses, and side effects of psychoactive drugs*, pp. 464–488. Freeman and Co, New York.

Kandel, E. (2006) *In Search of Memory: The Emergence of a New Science of Mind.* W. Norton & Co, New York.

Katzman, R., Terry, R., DeTeresa, R., Brown, T., Davies, P., Fuld, P., Renbing, X. & Peck, A. (1988) Clinical pathological and neurochemical changes in dementia: a subgroup with preserved mental status and numerous neocortical plaques. *Annals of Neurology*, **23**, 138–144.

Kelham, C. (2005) *Medicines Management Support Involving Assistive Technology.* Available at http://www.medicines-partnership.org/projects/current-projects/assistive-technology (accessed 27/02/06).

Kennedy, L., Neidlinger, S. & Scroggins, K. (1987) Effective compre-hensive discharge planning for hospitalized elderly. *The Gerontologist*, **27**, 577–580.

Kenney, W.L. & Chiu, P. (2001) Influence of age on thirst and fluid intake. *Medicine & Science in Sports & Exercise*, **33** (9), 1524–1532.

Keren, R. (2005) Managing Alzheimer's disease. *Elder Care: issues and options for Canadian physicians.* CMA Leadership Series. Canadian Medical Associa-tion, Ottowa.

Kester, L. & Stoller, J.K. (2003) Prevalence and causes of medication errors. *Clinical Pulmonary Medicine*, **10** (6), 322–326.

Kirkwood, T. (1999) *Time of Our Lives: The Science of Human Aging.* Oxford University Press, New York.

Kitzman, D.W. & Edwards, W.D. (1990) Age-related changes in the anatomy of the normal human heart. *Journal of Gerontology*, **45** (2), M33–M39.

Kitzman, D.W., Little, W.C., Brubaker, P.H., Anderson, R.T., Hundley, W.G., Marburger, C.T., Brosnihan, B., Morgan, T.M. & Stewart, K.P. (2002) Pathophysiological characterization of isolated diastolic heart failure in comparison to systolic heart failure. *Journal of the American Medical Association*, **288**, 2144–2150.

Knight, E.L. & Avorn, J. (2001) Quality indicators for appropriate medication use in vulnerable elders. *Annals of Internal Medicine*, **1355**, 703–710.

Knowles, M. (1990) *The Adult Learner. A Neglected Species*, 4th edn, pp. 18–50. Gulf Publishing Company, Texas.

Kolton, K.A. & Piccolo, P. (1988) Patient compliance: a challenge in practice. *Nurse Practitioner*, **13**, 37–50.

Koren, G. & Haslam, R.H. (1994) Pediatric medication errors: predicting and preventing tenfold error. *Journal of Clinical Pharmacology*, **34**, 1043–1045.

Krska, J., Cromarty, J.A., Arris, F., Jamieson, D., Hansford, D., Duffus, P.R., Downie, G. & Seymour, D.G. (2001) Pharmacist-led medication review in patients over 65: a randomised controlled trial in primary care. *Age and Ageing*, **30** (3), 205–211.

LaFerla, F.M. (2006) An array of genes implicated in Alzheimer's disease. *Neurobiology of Ageing*, **27**, 1078–1080.

Lahdenperä, T.S. & Kyngäs, H.A. (2000) Compliance and its evaluation in patents with hypertension. *Journal of Clinical Nursing*, **9**, 826–833.

Lakatta, E.G. & Sollot, S.J. (2002) The 'Heartbreak' of Older Age. *Molecular Interventions*, **2** (7), 431–446.

Lamy, P. (1990) Clinical Pharmacology issue of *Clinics in Geriatric Medicine*. W.B. Saunders, Philadelphia.

Landfield, P. (1988) Hippocampal neurobiological mechanisms of age related memory dysfunction. *Neurobiology of Aging*, **9**, 571–579.

Landis, S.J. (1990) Azithioprine or azidothymidine. *CMAJ*, **143** (7), 611.

Lang, A. & Lozano, A. (1998) Parkinson's Disease. *The New England Journal of Medicine*, **339** (16), 1130–1143.

Larsson, E., Kukull, W. & Buchner, D. (1987) Adverse drug reactions associated with global cognitive impairment in elderly persons. *Annals of Internal Medicine*, **107**, 169–173.

Latter, S., Rycroft-Malone, J., Yerrell, P. & Shaw, D. (2000) Evaluating educational preparation for a health education role in practice: the case of medication education. *Journal of Advanced Nursing*, **32**, 1282–1290.

Leape, L.L. (1994) Error in Medicine. *JAMA*, **278**, 1851–1857.

Leape, L.L., Brennan T.A. & Laird, N. (1991) The nature of adverse events in hospitalized patients. Results of the Harvard Medical Practice Study II. *New England Journal of Medicine*, **324**, 377–84.

Leipzig, R. (1999) Pharmacology and appropriate prescribing. In: Cobbs, E.L., Duthie, E.H.Jr. & Murphy, J.B. (eds). *Geriatrics review syllabus*, 4th edn, pp. 30–35. Kendall/Hunt, Dubuque, IA.

Leipzig, R.M. (2000) Keys to maximising benefit while avoiding adverse effects. *Geriatrics*, **56**, 30–34.

Lesar, T.S. (1992) Common prescribing errors. *Annals of Internal Medicine*, **117**, 537–8.

Lesar, T.S. (2002) Prescribing errors involving medication dosage forms. *Journal of General Internal Medicine*, **17** (8), 579–587.

Lesar, T.S., Briceland, L. & Stein, D. (1997) Medication-prescribing errors in a teaching hospital. A 19-year experience. *Archives of International Medicine*, **157**, 1569–1576.

Lewis, G. (2005) *Virtual Community Wards*. Presentation at Long Term Conditions – Predictive Case Finding Tool Conference, 27/10/05, Novotel London West, Hammersmith.

Lindley, C.M. & Tulley, M.P. (1992) Inappropriate medication is a major cause of adverse drug reactions in elderly people. *Age and Aging*, **21**, 294–300.

Livingstone, S. (2003) The Older Patient. *The Pharmaceutical Journal*, **270**, 862–863.

Lomaestro, B.M., Lesar, T.S. & Hagar, T.P. (1992) Errors in prescribing methotrexate. *JAMA*, **268** (15), 2031–2032.

LOPSDP (2003) Medicines Management Pilot. Executive Summary. The London Older People's Services Development Programme

Lowe, C.J., Raynor, D.K., Purvis, J., Farrin, A. & Hudson, J. (2000) Effects of medicine review and education programme for older people in general practice. *British Journal of Clinical Pharmacology*, **50**, 172–175.

Lowry, D.A. (1998) Issues of non-compliance in mental health. *Journal of Advanced Nursing*, **28**, 280–287.

Luke, R.G. & Beck, L.H. (1999) Gerontologizing nephrology. *Journal of the American Society of Nephrology*, **10**, 1824–1827.

Lustig, A. (2000) Medication error prevention by pharmacists – an Israeli solution. *Pharmacy World and Science*, **22**, 21–25.

Lutener, S. (2001) Legal framework of the GP/Pharmacist interface. *Prescriber*, **19**, 73–81.

Mackie, C.A., Lawson, D.H., Campbell, A., Maclaren, A.G. & Waigh, R. (1999) A randomised controlled trial of medication review in patients receiving polypharmacy in general practice. *Pharmaceutical Journal*, **263**, (suppl.) R7.

Mahdy, H.A. & Seymour, D.G. (1990) How much can elderly patients tell us about their medications? *Postgraduate Medical Journal*, **66**, 116–121.

Malinow, R. & Malenka, R. (2002) AMPA receptor trafficking and synaptic plasticity. *Annual Review of Neuroscience*, **25**, 103–126.

Mandelkow, E., Stamer, K., Vogel, R., Thies, E. & Mandelkow, E. (2003) Clogging of axons by tau, inhibition of axonal traffic and starvation of synapses. *Neurobiology of Ageing*, **24** (8), 1079–85.

Manias, E. & Bullock, S. (2002) The educational preparation of undergraduate nursing students in pharmacology: clinical nurses' perceptions and experiences of graduate nurses' medication knowledge. *International Journal of Nursing Studies*, **39**, 773–784.

Mannaesse, C.K. (1997) Adverse drug reactions in elderly patients as a contributing factor for hospital admission: cross sectional study. *BMJ*, **315**, 1057–1058.

Markham, J.A, McKian, K,P. Stroup, T.S. and Jurasca, J.M. (2005) Sexually dimorphic aging of dendritic morphology in CA1 of hippocampus. *Hippocampus*, **14**, 97–103.

Martens, K.H. (1998) An ethnographic study of the process of medication discharge education (MDE). *Journal of Advanced Nursing*, **27**, 341–348.

Mayor, S. (2001) NHS introduces new patient safety agency. *British Medical Journal*, **322**, 1013.

McLean, A.J., Cogger, V.C., Chong, G.C., Warren, A., Markus, A.M.A, Dahlstrom, J.E. & Le Couteur, D.G. (2003) Age-related pseudocapillarization of the human liver. *Journal of Pathology*, **200** (1), 112–117.

McLean, A.J. & LeCouteur, D.G. (2004) Aging biology and geriatric clinical pharmacology. *Pharmacological Reviews*, **56**, 163–184.

Medicines Partnership *Medicines Partnership From Compliance To Concordance Vision and Mission*. Available from http://www.medicines-partnership. org/index.asp?pgid=839 (accessed 27/2/06).

Medicines Partnership (2002) Medication Management. http://www. medicines-partnership-review/singleassessment/sap_med. http://www. managingmedicines. com/resource

Melk, A. & Halloran, P.F. (2001) Cell senescence and its implications for nephrology. *Journal of the American Society of Nephrology*, **12**, 385–393.

Mental Health Foundation (2001) Medicines and good health. A report on a UK survey of the availability of community based pharmaceutical care for older people with mental health needs. *Updates*, **3** (8), 1—6.

Mental Health Foundation (2004) Medicines and Drugs. Pharmaceutical Care Services for Older People with Mental Health Problems Living in the Community. www.Mhilli.org/medicines/rptpahrmsum.htm.

Merck (2005) *The Merck Manual of Geriatrics*, 3rd edn, editor-in-chief, M.H. Beers, Chapter 102, Aging and The Gastrointestinal Tract. Accessed online at http://www.merck.com/mrkshared/mmg/sec13/ch102/ch102h.jsp (19/6/06).

Mezey, E. (2003) Hepatic, biliary and pancreatic disease. In: Hazzard, W.R., Andres, R., Bierman, E.L. & Blass, J.P. (eds) *Principles of Geriatric Medicine and Gerontology*, 5th edn, pp. 601–612.

Milburn, A. (2001) Secretary of State for Health. Forward in: *National Service Framework (NSF) for Older People*. Department of Health, London.

Miletic, D., Fuckar, Z., Sustic, A., Mozetic, V., Stimac, D. & Zauhar, G. (1998) Sonographic measurement of absolute and relative renal length in adults. *Journal of Clinical Ultrasound*, **26**, 185–189.

Moore, A., Hawkey, C.J. & Emery, P. (2001) Prescribing in the UK. *The Lancet*, **357**, 809–810.

Moore, N., Lecointre, D., Noblet, C. & Mabille, M. (1998) Frequency and cost of serious adverse drug reactions in a department of general medicine. *British Journal of Clinical Pharmacology*, **45**, 301–308.

Morgan, J.D., Wright, D.J. & Chrysyn, H. (2000) Comparison of pharmacist run medication review clinics using different patient selection criteria. *Pharmaceutical Journal*, **265**, R28.

Morris, J., Beaumont, D. & Oliver, D. (2006) Decent health care for older people. *BMJ*, **332**, 1166–1168.

Muir, A., Sanders, L.L., Williams, M.S., Wilkinson, E. & Schamader, K. (2001) Reducing medication regimen complexity. A controlled trial. *Journal of General Internal Medicine*, **16**, 77–82.

Mula, C. (2006) Nurse prescribing reaches new horizons. *International Journal of Palliative Nursing*, **12** (2), 52–55.

Mullen, P.D. (1997) Compliance becomes concordance. *British Medical Journal*, **314**, 691.

Nathan, C. (2002. Points of control in inflammation. *Nature*, **420**, 846–852.

National Centre for Complementary and Alternative Medicine (2004) *St John's Wort and the Treatment of Depression*. Available from http://ncam.nih.Gov/health/stjohnswort/ (accessed January 2006).

National Coordinating Council for Medication Error Reporting and Prevention (2002) Consumer information for safe medication use. www.nccmerp.org/consumerinfo.html (accessed 23 February 2004).

National Health Service (2002) Northern Yorkshire Regional Office. North Yorkshire Primary Care Trust.

Naugler, C.T. (2000) Development and validation of an improving prescribing in the elderly tool. *Canadian Journal of Clinical Pharmacology*, **7**, 301–307.

Neary, J. (2002) Clinical medication review by pharmacists would improve care. *BMJ*, **324** (7736), 548.

NHS Connecting for Health (2006) *The Electronic Prescription Service*. Available at http://www.connectingforhealth.nhs.uk/eps (accessed 27/02/2006).

NICE (2002) *Inherited Clinical Guideline G; Management of Type 2 Diabetes – Management of Blood Glucose*. National Institute for Health and Clinical Excellence, London.

NPA (1998) *Medication Management: Everybody's Problem*. The National Pharmaceutical Association, St Albans.

NPC (2003) Modernising Medicines Management Guide. www.npc.co.uk/npc_pubs.htm. National Prescribing Centre, Liverpool.

NPSA (2003) A British Medical Journal study into the frequency of adverse drug reactions. http://www.81.144.177.110/web/display?contentld=3097 (accessed 23 February 2004). National Patient Safety Agency, London.

NPSA (2004) Methotrexate alert. http://www.npsa.org.uk. National Patient Safety Agency, London.

Nurse Practitioner (2001) editorial. Safe prescribing. Nurse practitioner. *American Journal of Primary Health Care*, **26** (6), 60.

Nytanga, B. (1997) Psychosocial theories of patient non-compliance. *Professional Nurse*, **12**, 331–334.

Oboh, L. (2006) Pharmacists can help improve older people's medicines management. *The Pharmaceutical Journal*, **276**, 206–207.

Office of Population Censuses and Surveys (OPCS) (1996). *Living in Britain: Results from the 1994 General Household Survey*. HMSO, London.

O'Mahony, S. (2000) Pharmacokinetics. In: Crome, P., Ford, G. (eds) *Drugs and the Older Population*, pp. 58–89. Imperial College Press, London.

Opdycke, R.A.C., Ascione, F.J., Shimp, L.A. & Rosen, R.I. (1992) A systematic approach to educating elderly patients about their medications. *Patient Education and Counselling*, **19**, 43–60.

Osborne, C.A. & Batty, G. (1997) Development of prescribing indicators for elderly medical inpatients. *British Journal of Clinical Pharmacology*, **43**, 91–97.

O'Shea, E. (1999) Factors contributing to medication errors; a literature review. *Journal of Clinical Nursing*, **8**, (5), 496–504.

Papastrat, K. & Wallace, S. (2003) Teaching Baccalaureate nursing students to prevent medication errors using a problem-based learning approach. *Journal of Nurse Education*, **42**, 459–464.

Pape, T.M. (2001) Searching for the final answer: factors contributing to medication administration errors. *The Journal of Continuing Education in Nursing*, **32**, 152–160.

Patsdaughter, C.A. & Pesznecker, B.L. (1988) Medication regimens and the elderly home care client. *Journal of Gerontological Nursing*, **14**, 30–34.

Pawelec, G., Hirokawa, K. & Fulop, T. (2001). Altered T-cell signalling in ageing. *Mechanisms of Ageing and Development*, **122**, 1613–1617.

Pearson, B., Skelly, T., Wileman, D. & Masud, T. (2002) Unplanned readmission to hospital: a comparison of the views of general practitioners and hospital staff. *Age and Ageing*, **31** (2), 141–143.

Peck, C. (1985) *Bedside Clinical Pharmacokinetics*. Pharmacometric Press, Rockville, MD.

Petty, D., Rayner, D.K., Zermansky, A. & Alldred, D. (2005) Medication review by pharmacists – the evidence still suggests benefit. *Pharmaceutical Journal*, **274**, 618–619.

Polifroni, E.C. (2002) Medication errors: more basic than a system issue. *Journal of Nurse Education*, **42**, 455–458.

Porter, P., Pandya, Y., et al. (2004) Cortical cholinergic deficit is associated with plaque development at preclinical stages of Alzheimer's disease. *Neurobiology of Ageing*, **25** (S2), 79.

Proos, M., Reiley, P, Eagon, J., Stengrevices, S., Castile, J. & Aarion, D. (1992) A study of the effects of self-medication on patients' knowledge of and compliance with their medication regime. *Journal of Nursing Care Quality*, (special report), 18–26.

PSNC (2007) Pharmaceutical Services Negotiating Committee, Medicines Use Review Service Specification. http://www.psnc.org.uk/index.php?type=page&pid=107&k=2 (accessed 29/01/07)

Pullar, T., Roach, P. & Mellor, E.J. (1989). Patients' knowledge concerning their medications on discharge from hospital. *Journal of Clinical Pharmacy and Therapeutics*, **14**, 57–59.

Randles, A. & Black, P. (1999) An investigation into the role of a practice pharmacist in the processing of discharge medication in one GP practice. *Pharmacy Journal*, **263**, R65.

Rang, H., Dale, M.M. & Ritter, S. (2000) *Pharmacology*. Churchill Livingstone, Edinburgh.

RCGP (2000) *The RCGP's view on the future role of the pharmacist in primary care.* Royal College of General Practitioners, London.

RCP (1997) *Medication for older people.* A report of the Royal College of Physicians, London.

Reddy, P. & McWeeney, S. (2006) Mapping cellular transcriptosomes in autopsied Alzheimer's disease subjects and relevant animal models. *Neurobiology of Ageing*, **27**, 1060–1070.

Redfern, S.J. (1991) *Nursing Elderly People*, 2nd edn. Churchill Livingstone, Edinburgh.

Redfern, S. & Ross, F. (2006) *Nursing Older People*, 4th edn. Churchill Livingstone Elsevier, London.

Rehman, H.U. (2004) Pharmacotherapy in old age. *Journal of the Royal College of Physicians of Edinburgh*, **34**, 21–27.

Reid, J. (2005) Health Secretary cited in Beasley C. *Community Matrons will make a difference to patients' lives – Chief Nursing Officer press release.* Department of Health, London.

Rich, M.W., Gray, D.B., Beckham, V., Wittenberg, C. & Luther, P. (1996) Effect of a multidisciplinary intervention on medication compliance in elderly patient with congestive heart failure. *The American Journal of Medicine*, **101**, 270–276.

Ridely, S.A., Booth, S.A. & Thompson, C.M. (2004) Prescription errors in UK critical care units. *Anaesthesia*, **29** (12), 1193–1200.

Rideout, S., Waters, W.E. & George, C.F. (1986) Knowledge of and attitudes to medicines in the Southampton community. *British Journal of Clinical Pharmacology*, **212**, 701–712.

Roberson, M.H.B. (1992) The meaning of compliance: patient perspectives. *Quality Health Review*, **2**, 7–26.

Roberts, J. & Tumer, N. (1988) Pharmacodynamic basis for altered drug action in the elderly. *Clinics in Geriatric Medicine*, **4**, 127–149.

Rochon, P.A. & Gurwitz, J.H. (1999) Prescribing for seniors: neither too much nor too little. *JAMA*, **282**, 113–115.

Rodwell, G.E.J., Sonu, R., Zahn, J.M., Lund, J. & Wilhelmy J. (2004) A transcriptional profile of aging in the human kidney. *Public Library of Science Biology*, **2** (12), 2191–2201.

Rolfe, S. & Harper, N. (1995) Ability of hospital doctors to calculate drug dosages. *BMJ*, **310** (6988), 1173–1174.

RPSGB (2001) *The Administration and Control of Medicines in Care Homes.* Royal Pharmaceutical Society of Great Britain, London.

RPSGB (2003) *Pharmacy in the Future: Medicines Management.* http://www.rpsgb.org.uk/nhsplan/medman.htm. Royal Pharmaceutical Society for Great Britain, London.

RPSGB/Merck Sharp & Dohme (1996) 'Partnership in Medicine Taking: A consultation document.' Royal Pharmaceutical Society of Great Britain, London.

RSPGB/Merck Sharp & Dohme (1997) 'From Compliance to Concordance: Achieving Shared Goals in Medicine Taking.' Royal Pharmaceutical Society of Great Britain, London.

Rudd, P. (1993) Partial compliance: implications for clinical practice. *Journal of Cardiovascular Pharmacology*, **22**, Suppl. A, S1–5.

Rudd, P., Ahmed, S., Zachary, V., Barton, C. & Bonduelle, D. (1992) Issues in patient compliance: the search for therapeutic sufficiency. *Cardiology*, **80**, Suppl. 1, 2–10.

Rutten, B., van der Kolt, N., Schaefer, S., van Zandvoort, M., Bayer, T. Steinbusch, H. et al. (2005) Age related loss of synaptophysin-immunoreactive presynaptic boutons within the hippocampus of APP751SL, PS1M146L and APP751SL/PS1M146L transgenic mice. *American Journal of Pathology*, **167**, 161–173.

Ryan, A.A. & Chambers, M. (2000) Medication management and older patients: an individualized and systematic approach. *Journal of Clinical Nursing*, **9**, 732–741.

Sabbagh, M., Farlow, M., Relkin, N. & Beach, T. (2006) Do cholinergic therapies have disease modifying effects in Alzheimer's disease. *Alzheimer's and Dementia*, **2** (2), 118–125.

Safwat, M. & Goodyer, L. (2005) Reflections on HOMER: A hospital-based discharge medication review scheme 2005. *International Journal of Pharmacy Practice*, **13**, (suppl.) R31.

Sampson, E.L., Gould, V., Lee, D. & Blanchard, B. (2006) Differences in care received by patients with and without dementia who died during acute hospital admission: a retrospective case study. *Age and Ageing*, **35**, 187–189.

Schmucker, D.L. (1998) Aging and the liver: an update. *Journals of Gerontology Series A: Biological Sciences and Medical Sciences*, **53** (5), B315–B320.

Schmucker, D.L. (2001) Liver function and phase I drug metabolism in the elderly: a paradox. *Drugs & Aging*, **18** (11), 837–851.

Schwartz, J.B. (1999) Clinical pharmacology. In: Hazzard, W.R., Blass, J.P., Ettinger, W.H. Jr. (eds) *Principles of Geriatric Medicine and Gerontology*, 4th edn, pp. 303–331. McGraw Hill, New York.

Schweizer, A.K. & Hughes, C. (2001) Nursing and residential care for the elderly in Northern Ireland: the contributions of the pharmacist. *Pharmacy World & Science*, **23** (5), 195–199.

SCIE (2005) SCIE Research briefing 15: Helping older people to take prescribed medication in their own home: what works? http://www.scie.org.uk/publications/briefings/briefing15/index.asp. Social Care Institute for Excellence, London.

Sheehan, O. & Feely, J. (1999) Prescribing considerations in elderly patients. *Prescriber*, **10**, 75–83.

Shelton, P.S. (2000) Assessing medication appropriateness in the elderly: a review of available measures. *Drugs and Ageing*, **16** (6), 437–450.

Smith, M., Sayre, L., Monnier, G. & Perry, G. (1995) Radical AGEing in Alzheimer's disease. *Trends in Neuroscience*, **18**, 172–176.

Stamer, K., Vogel, R., Thies, E., Mandelkow, E. & Mandelkow, E.M, (2002) Tau blocks traffic of organelles, neurofilaments, and APP vesicles in neurons and enhances oxidative stress. *Journal of Cell Biology*, **156** (96), 1051–1063.

Stimson, G.V. (1974) Obeying doctor's orders: a view from the other side. *Social Science and Medicine*, **8**, 97–104.

Sultana, R., Boyd-Kimball, D., Poon, H., Cai, J., Pierce, W., Klein, J., Markesbery, W., Zhou, X., Lu, K. & Butterfield, D. (2006) Oxidative modification of Pin 1 in Alzheimer's disease hippocampus: A redox proteomics analysis. *Neurobiology of Ageing*, **27**, 918–925.

Sultana, R. & Butterfield, D. (2004) Oxidatively modified GST and MRPI in Alzheimer's disease brain, implications for accumulation of reactive lipid peroxidation products. *Neurochemistry Research*, **279** (29), 2215–2220.

Swift, C.G. (2001) Care of older people: Falls in later life and their consequences – implementing effective services. *British Medical Journal*, **322**, 855–857.

Swift, C.G. (2003) The clinical pharmacology of ageing. *British Journal of Clinical Pharmacology*, **56** (3), 249–253.

Syred, M.E.J. (1981) The abdication of the role of health education by hospital nurses. *Journal of Advanced Nursing*, **6**, 27–33.

Taffet, G.E. (1999) Age-related physiological changes. In: Cobbs, E.L., Duthie, E.H.Jr., Murphy, J.B. (eds) *Geriatrics Review Syllabus*, 4th edn, pp. 10–23. Kendall/Hunt, Dubuque. IA.

Taffet, G.E. & Lakatta, E.G. (1999) Aging of the cardiovascular system. In: Hazzard, W.R., Andres, R., Bierman, E.L., Blass, J.P., Ettinger, W.H., Halter, J.B. & Ouslander, J.G. (eds) *Principles of Geriatric Medicine and Gerontology*. McGraw-Hill, New York.

Taunton, R.L., Kleinbeck, S.V.M., Stafford, R., Woods, C.Q. & Bott, M.J. (1994) Patient outcomes. Are they linked to registered nurse absenteeism, separation, or work load? *Journal of Nursing Administration*, **24** (4), 48–55.

Teichman, P. (2001) Reducing medication errors. *JAMA*, **286** (17), 2092.

Thompson, S. & Crome, P. (2002) Appropriate prescribing in older people. *Reviews in Clinical Gerontology*, **12**, 213–220.

Tian, Y., Serino, R. & Verbalis, J.G. (2004) Downregulation of renal vasopressin V2 receptor and aquaporin-2 expression parallels age-associated defects in urine concentration. *American Journal of Physiology – Renal Physiology*, **287** (4), F797–F805.

Tight, M. (1998) *Key Concepts in Adult Education and Training*, 2nd edn, pp. 23–45. Routledge, New York.

Timiras, P. (2002) The gastrointestinal tract and liver. In: Timiras, P. (ed.) *Physiological Basis of Aging and Geriatrics*, 3rd edn, pp. 359–374. CRC Press, Boca Raton, FL.

Timiras, M.L. & Leary, J. (2002) The kidney, the lower urinary tract, body fluids and the prostate. In: Timiras, P. *Physiological Basis of Aging and Geriatrics*, 3rd edn, pp. 337–358. CRC Press. Boca Raton, FL.

Toescu, E.C., Verkhratsky, A. & Landfield, P. (2004) Ca^{2+} regulation and gene expression in normal brain aging. *Trends in Neuroscience*, **27**, 614–620.

Trinkle, R. & Wu, J.K. (1997) Sources of medication errors involving paediatric chemotherapy patients, *Hospital Pharmacy*, **32**, 853–859.

Tulip, S. & Campbell, D. (2001) Evaluating pharmaceutical care in hospital. *Hospital Pharmacist*, **8**, 275–279.

Uemura, E. (1985) Age related changes in the subiculum of *Macac mulatto*; synaptic density. *Experimental Neurology*, **87**, 403–411.

Unutzer, J., Rubenstein. L., Katon, W., Tang, L., Duan, N., Lagomasino, I. & Wells, K. (2001) Two year effects of quality improvement on medication management of depression. *Archives General Psychiatry*, **58** (1), 935–942.

Vincent, G., Neale, G. & Woloshynowych, M. (2001) Adverse events in British hospitals: preliminary retrospective record review. *BMJ*, **322** (7285), 517–519.

Wagnild, G. & Grupp, K. (1991) Major stresses among elderly home care clients. *Home Healthcare Nurse*, **9**, 15–21.

Walker, J. & Wynne, H.A. (1999) The frequency and severity of adverse drug reactions in elderly people. *Age and Ageing*, **23**, 255–259.

Walkin, L. (2000) *Teaching and Learning in Further and Adult Education*, 2nd edn, pp.18–34. Stanley Thornes, Cheltenham.

Walley, T. & Scott, A.K. (1995) Prescribing in the elderly. *Postgraduate Medical Journal*, **71**, 466–471.

Webb, C., Addison, C., Holman, H., Saklaki, B. & Wagner, A. (1990) Self-medication for elderly patients. *Nursing Times*, **86**, 46–49.

Weinman, J. (1990) Providing written information for patients: psychological considerations. *Journal of the Royal Society of Medicine*, **83**, 292–297.

Wiggins, J. (2003) Changes in renal function. In: Hazzard, W.R., Blass, J.P., Halter, J.B., Ouslander, J.G. & Tinetti, M.E. (eds) *Principles of Geriatric Medicine and Gerontology*, 5th edn, pp. 543–549. McGraw Hill, New York.

Williams, E.I. & Fitton, F. (1988) Factors affecting early unplanned readmission of elderly patients to hospital. *BMJ*, **297**, 784–787.

Winland-Brown, J.E. & Valiante, J. (2000) Effectiveness of different medication management approaches on elders' medication adherence. *Outcomes Management for Nursing Practice*, **4**, 172–176.

Winslow, E.H. (1976) The role of the nurse in patient education, focus the cardiac patient. *Nursing Clinics of North America*, **11**, 213–222.

Wolock, I., Schlesinger, E., Dinerman, M. & Seaton, R. (1987) The posthospital needs and care of patients: implications for discharge planning. *Social Work in Health Care*, **12**, 61–76.

Woodhouse, K.W. & Wynne, H.A. (1992) The pharmacology of aging. In: Brocklehurst, J.C., Tallis, R.C. & Fillit, H.M. (eds) *Textbook of Geriatric Medicine and Gerontology*, 4th edn, pp. 23–46. Churchill Livingstone, London.

Wright, D. (2002) Tablet crushing is a widespread practice but it is not safe and may not be legal. *Pharmaceutical Journal*, **269**, 132.

Zermansky, A.G. (1996) Who controls repeats? *British Journal of General Practice*, **46**, 643–647.

Zermansky, A.G., Petty, D.R., Raynor, D.K., Freemantle, N., Vail, A. & Lowe, C.J. (2001) Randomised controlled trial of clinical medication review by a pharmacist of elderly patients receiving repeat prescriptions in general practice. *BMJ*, **323**, 1340–1343.

Zhu, X., Raina, A., Lee, H., Casadesus, G., Smith, M. & Perry, G. (2004) Oxidative stress signalling in Alzheimer's disease. *Brain Research*, **1000**, 32–39.

Zimmermann, P.G. & Cousins, D. (2004) Decreasing drug errors. *Journal of Emergency Nursing*, **30** (4), 359.

Index